Virtual Clinical Excursions—

for

Lowdermilk, Perry, Cashion, and Alden:
Maternity & Women's Health Care
11th Edition

prepared by

Kelly Ann Crum, RN, MSN
Chair, Department of Nursing
Associate Professor of Nursing
Maranatha Baptist Bible College
Watertown, Wisconsin

software developed by

Wolfsong Informatics, LLC
Tucson, Arizona

ELSEVIER
MOSBY

ELSEVIER
MOSBY

3251 Riverport Lane
Maryland Heights, Missouri 63043

Notice

Knowledge and best practice in this field are constantly changing. As new research and experience broaden our understanding, changes in research methods, professional practices, or medical treatment may become necessary.

Practitioners and researchers must always rely on their own experience and knowledge in evaluating and using any information, methods, compounds, or experiments described herein. In using such information or methods they should be mindful of their own safety and the safety of others, including parties for whom they have a professional responsibility.

With respect to any drug or pharmaceutical products identified, readers are advised to check the most current information provided (i) on procedures featured or (ii) by the manufacturer of each product to be administered, to verify the recommended dose or formula, the method and duration of administration, and contraindications. It is the responsibility of practitioners, relying on their own experience and knowledge of their patients, to make diagnoses, to determine dosages and the best treatment for each individual patient, and to take all appropriate safety precautions.

To the fullest extent of the law, neither the Publisher nor the authors, contributors, or editors, assume any liability for any injury and/or damage to persons or property as a matter of products liability, negligence or otherwise, or from any use or operation of any methods, products, instructions, or ideas contained in the material herein.

ISBN: 978-0-323-37720-1

Printed in the United States of America

Last digit is the print number: 9 8 7 6 5 4 3 2 1

Workbook prepared by

Kelly Ann Crum, RN, MSN
Chair, Department of Nursing
Associate Professor of Nursing
Maranatha Baptist Bible College
Watertown, Wisconsin

Previous edition prepared by

Kim D. Cooper, RN, MSN
Ivy Tech Community College
Terre Haute, Indiana

Textbook

Deitra Leonard Lowdermilk, RNC, PhD, FAAN
Clinical Professor Emerita, School of Nursing
University of North Carolina at Chapel Hill
Chapel Hill, North Carolina

Shannon E. Perry, RN, PhD, FAAN
Professor Emerita, School of Nursing
San Francisco State University
San Francisco, California

Kitty Cashion, RN, BC, MSN
Clinical Nurse Specialist
Department of Obstetrics and Gynecology
Division of Maternal-Fetal Medicine
University of Tennessee Health Science Center
Memphis, Tennessee

Kathryn Rhodes Alden, RN, MSN, EdD, IBCLC
Clinical Associate Professor, School of Nursing
University of North Carolina at Chapel Hill
Chapel Hill, North Carolina

Contents

Table of Contents
Lowdermilk, Perry, Cashion, and Alden:
Maternity & Women's Health Care, 11th Edition

GETTING SET UP WITH VCE ONLINE

The product you have purchased is part of the Evolve Learning System. Please read the following information thoroughly to get started.

■ HOW TO ACCESS YOUR VCE RESOURCES ON EVOLVE

There are two ways to access your VCE Resources on Evolve:

1. If your instructor has enrolled you in your VCE Evolve Resources, you will receive an email with your registration details.

2. If your instructor has asked you to self-enroll in your VCE Evolve Resources, he or she will provide you with your Course ID (for example, 1479_jdoe73_0001). You will then need to follow the instructions at https://evolve.elsevier.com/cs/studentEnroll.html.

■ HOW TO ACCESS THE ONLINE VIRTUAL HOSPITAL

The online virtual hospital is available through the Evolve VCE Resources. There is no software to download or install: the online virtual hospital runs within your Internet browser, using a pop-up window.

■ TECHNICAL REQUIREMENTS

- Broadband connection (DSL or cable)
- 1024 x 768 screen resolution
- Mozilla Firefox 18.0, Internet Explorer 9.0, Google Chrome, or Safari 5 (or higher)
  Note: Pop-up blocking software/settings must be disabled.
- Adobe Acrobat Reader
- Additional technical requirements available at http://evolvesupport.elsevier.com

■ HOW TO ACCESS THE WORKBOOK

There are two ways to access the workbook portion of *Virtual Clinical Excursions:*

1. Print workbook
2. An electronic version of the workbook, available within the VCE Evolve Resources

■ TECHNICAL SUPPORT

Technical support for *Virtual Clinical Excursions* is available by visiting the Technical Support Center at http://evolvesupport.elsevier.com or by calling 1-800-222-9570 inside the United States and Canada.

Trademarks: Windows® and Macintosh® are registered trademarks.

A QUICK TOUR

Welcome to *Virtual Clinical Excursions—Obstetrics*, a virtual hospital setting in which you can work with multiple complex patient simulations and also learn to access and evaluate the information resources that are essential for high-quality patient care. The virtual hospital, Pacific View Regional Hospital, has realistic architecture and access to patient rooms, a Nurses' Station, and a Medication Room.

■ BEFORE YOU START

Make sure you have your textbook nearby when you use *Virtual Clinical Excursions*. You will want to consult topic areas in your textbook frequently while working with the virtual hospital and workbook.

■ HOW TO SIGN IN

- Enter your name on the Student Nurse identification badge.
- Now choose one of the four periods of care in which to work. In Periods of Care 1 through 3, you can actively engage in patient assessment, entry of data in the electronic patient record (EPR), and medication administration. Period of Care 4 presents the day in review. Click on the appropriate period of care. (For this quick tour, choose **Period of Care 1: 0730-0815**.)
- This takes you to the Patient List screen (see the *How to Select a Patient* section below). Note that the virtual time is provided in the box at the lower left corner of the screen (0730, since we chose Period of Care 1).

Note: If you choose to work during Period of Care 4: 1900-2000, the Patient List screen is skipped since you are not able to visit patients or administer medications during the shift. Instead, you are taken directly to the Nurses' Station, where the records of all the patients on the floor are available for your review.

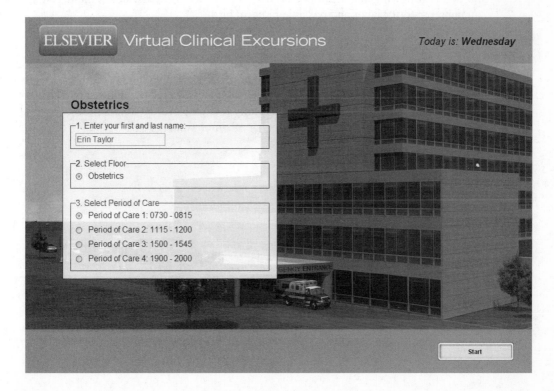

■ PATIENT LIST

OBSTETRICS UNIT

Dorothy Grant (Room 201)
30-week intrauterine pregnancy—A 25-year-old multipara Caucasian female admitted with abdominal trauma following a domestic violence incident. Her complications include preterm labor and extensive social issues such as acquiring safe housing for her family upon discharge.

Stacey Crider (Room 202)
27-week intrauterine pregnancy—A 21-year-old primigravida Native American female admitted for intravenous tocolysis, bacterial vaginosis, and poorly controlled insulin-dependent gestational diabetes. Strained family relationships and social isolation complicate this patient's ability to comply with strict dietary requirements and prenatal care.

Kelly Brady (Room 203)
26-week intrauterine pregnancy—A 35-year-old primigravida Caucasian female urgently admitted for progressive symptoms of preeclampsia. A history of inadequate coping with major life stressors leave her at risk for a recurrence of depression as she faces a diagnosis of HELLP syndrome and the delivery of a severely premature infant.

Maggie Gardner (Room 204)
22-week intrauterine pregnancy—A 41-year-old multigravida African-American female admitted for a high risk pregnancy evaluation and rule out diagnosis of systemic lupus erythematosus. Coping with chronic pain, fatigue, and a history of multiple miscarriages contribute to an anxiety disorder and the need for social service intervention.

Gabriela Valenzuela (Room 205)
34-week intrauterine pregnancy—A 21-year-old primigravida Hispanic female with a history of mitral valve prolapse admitted for uterine cramping and vaginal bleeding suggestive of placental abruption following an unrestrained motor vehicle accident. Her needs include staff support for an unprepared-for labor and possible preterm birth.

Laura Wilson (Room 206)
37-week intrauterine pregnancy—An 18-year-old primigravida Caucasian female urgently admitted after being found unconscious at home. Her complications include HIV-positive status and chronic polysubstance abuse. Unrealistic expectations of parenthood and living with a chronic illness combined with strained family relations prompt comprehensive social and psychiatric evaluations initiated on the day of simulation.

■ HOW TO SELECT A PATIENT

- You can choose one or more patients to work with from the Patient List by checking the box to the left of the patient name(s). For this quick tour, select Dorothy Grant. (In order to receive a scorecard for a patient, the patient must be selected before proceeding to the Nurses' Station.)
- Click on **Get Report** to the right of the medical records number (MRN) to view a summary of the patient's care during the 12-hour period before your arrival on the unit.
- After reviewing the report, click on **Go to Nurses' Station** in the right lower corner to begin your care. (*Note:* If you have been assigned to care for multiple patients, you can click on **Return to Patient List** to select and review the report for each additional patient before going to the Nurses' Station.)

Note: Even though the Patient List is initially skipped when you sign in to work for Period of Care 4, you can still access this screen if you wish to review the shift report for any of the patients. To do so, simply click on **Patient List** near the top left corner of the Nurses' Station (or click on the clipboard to the left of the Kardex). Then click on **Get Report** for the patient(s) whose care you are reviewing. This may be done during any period of care.

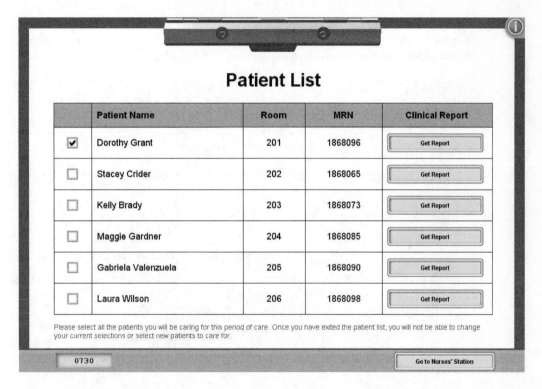

Patient List

	Patient Name	Room	MRN	Clinical Report
☑	Dorothy Grant	201	1868096	Get Report
☐	Stacey Crider	202	1868065	Get Report
☐	Kelly Brady	203	1868073	Get Report
☐	Maggie Gardner	204	1868085	Get Report
☐	Gabriela Valenzuela	205	1868090	Get Report
☐	Laura Wilson	206	1868098	Get Report

Please select all the patients you will be caring for this period of care. Once you have exited the patient list, you will not be able to change your current selections or select new patients to care for.

0730   Go to Nurses' Station

■ HOW TO FIND A PATIENT'S RECORDS

Nurses' Station

Within the Nurses' Station, you will see:

1. A clipboard that contains the patient list for that floor.
2. A chart rack with patient charts labeled by room number, a notebook labeled Kardex, and a notebook labeled MAR (Medication Administration Record).
3. A desktop computer with access to the Electronic Patient Record (EPR).
4. A tool bar across the top of the screen that can also be used to access the Patient List, EPR, Chart, MAR, and Kardex. This tool bar is also accessible from each patient's room.
5. A Drug Guide containing information about the medications you are able to administer to your patients.
6. A Laboratory Guide containing normal value ranges for all laboratory tests you may come across in the virtual patient hospital.
7. A tool bar across the bottom of the screen that can be used to access the Floor Map, patient rooms, Medication Room, and Drug Guide.

As you run your cursor over an item, it will be highlighted. To select, simply click on the item. As you use these resources, you will always be able to return to the Nurses' Station by clicking on the **Return to Nurses' Station** bar located in the right lower corner of your screen.

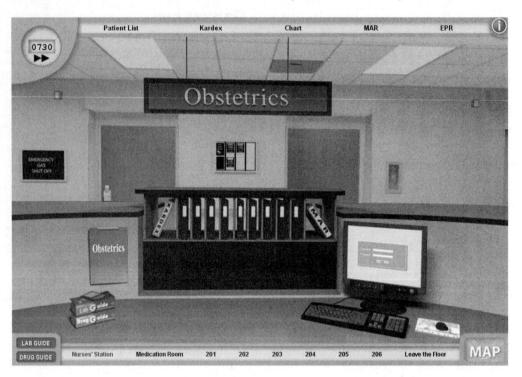

MEDICATION ADMINISTRATION RECORD (MAR)

The MAR icon located on the tool bar at the top of your screen accesses current 24-hour medications for each patient. Click on the icon and the MAR will open. (*Note:* You can also access the MAR by clicking on the MAR notebook on the far right side of the book rack in the center of the screen.) Within the MAR, tabs on the right side of the screen allow you to select patients by room number. Be careful to make sure you select the correct tab number for *your* patient rather than simply reading the first record that appears after the MAR opens. Each MAR sheet lists the following:

- Medications
- Route and dosage of each medication
- Times of administration of each medication

Note: The MAR changes each day. Expired MARs are stored in the patients' charts.

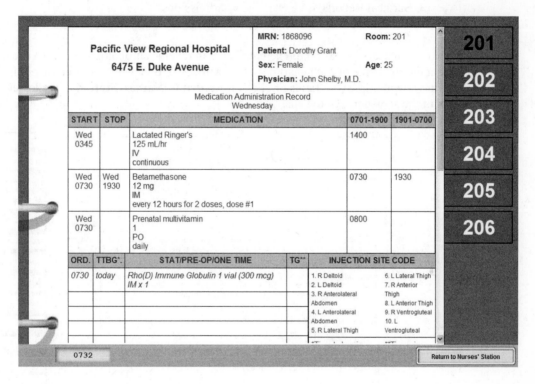

CHARTS

To access patient charts, either click on the **Chart** icon at the top of your screen or anywhere within the chart rack in the center of the Nurses' Station screen. When the close-up view appears, the individual charts are labeled by room number. To open a chart, click on the room number of the patient whose chart you wish to review. The patient's name and allergies will appear on the left side of the screen, along with a list of tabs on the right side of the screen, allowing you to view the following data:

- Allergies
- Physician's Orders
- Physician's Notes
- Nurse's Notes
- Laboratory Reports
- Diagnostic Reports
- Surgical Reports
- Consultations
- Patient Education
- History and Physical
- Nursing Admission
- Expired MARs
- Consents
- Mental Health
- Admissions
- Emergency Department

Information appears in real time. The entries are in reverse chronologic order, so use the down arrow at the right side of each chart page to scroll down to view previous entries. Flip from tab to tab to view multiple data fields or click on **Return to Nurses' Station** in the lower right corner of the screen to exit the chart.

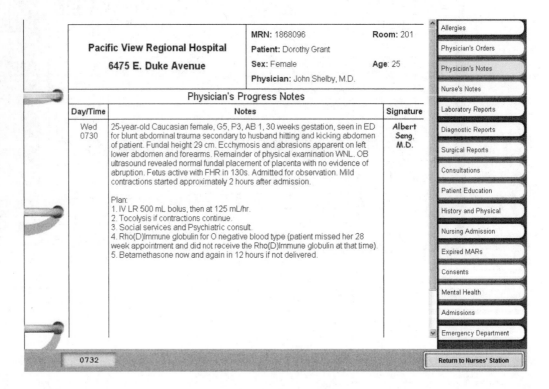

ELECTRONIC PATIENT RECORD (EPR)

The EPR can be accessed from the computer in the Nurses' Station or from the EPR icon located in the tool bar at the top of your screen. To access a patient's EPR:
- Click on either the computer screen or the **EPR** icon.
- Your username and password are automatically filled in.
- Click on **Login** to enter the EPR.
- *Note:* Like the MAR, the EPR is arranged numerically. Thus when you enter, you are initially shown the records of the patient in the lowest room number on the floor. To view the correct data for *your* patient, remember to select the correct room number, using the drop-down menu for the Patient field at the top left corner of the screen.

The EPR used in Pacific View Regional Hospital represents a composite of commercial versions being used in hospitals. You can access the EPR:
- to review existing data for a patient (by room number).
- to enter data you collect while working with a patient.

The EPR is updated daily, so no matter what day or part of a shift you are working, there will be a current EPR with the patient's data from the past days of the current hospital stay. This type of simulated EPR allows you to examine how data for different attributes have changed over time, as well as to examine data for all of a patient's attributes at a particular time. The EPR is fully functional (as it is in a real-life hospital). You can enter such data as blood pressure, breath sounds, and certain treatments. The EPR will not, however, allow you to enter data for a previous time period. Use the arrows at the bottom of the screen to move forward and backward in time.

Patient: 201		Category: Vital Signs				0735
Name: Dorothy Grant	Wed 0700	Wed 0715	Wed 0733		Code Meanings	
PAIN: LOCATION	A			A	Abdomen	
PAIN: RATING	1-2			Ar	Arm	
PAIN: CHARACTERISTICS	I			B	Back	
PAIN: VOCAL CUES				C	Chest	
PAIN: FACIAL CUES				Ft	Foot	
PAIN: BODILY CUES				H	Head	
PAIN: SYSTEM CUES				Hd	Hand	
PAIN: FUNCTIONAL EFFECTS				L	Left	
PAIN: PREDISPOSING FACTORS				Lg	Leg	
PAIN: RELIEVING FACTORS				Lw	Lower	
PCA				N	Neck	
TEMPERATURE (F)	98.2			NN	See Nurses notes	
TEMPERATURE (C)				OS	Operative site	
MODE OF MEASUREMENT	O			Or	See Physicians orders	
SYSTOLIC PRESSURE	126			PN	See Progress notes	
DIASTOLIC PRESSURE	68			R	Right	
BP MODE OF MEASUREMENT	NIBP			Up	Upper	
HEART RATE	70					
RESPIRATORY RATE	18					
SpO2 (%)	96					
BLOOD GLUCOSE						
WEIGHT						
HEIGHT						

Return to Nurses' Station

At the top of the EPR screen, you can choose patients by their room numbers. In addition, you have access to 17 different categories of patient data. To change patients or data categories, click the down arrow to the right of the room number or category.

The categories of patient data in the EPR are as follows:

- Vital Signs
- Respiratory
- Cardiovascular
- Neurologic
- Gastrointestinal
- Excretory
- Musculoskeletal
- Integumentary
- Reproductive
- Psychosocial
- Wounds and Drains
- Activity
- Hygiene and Comfort
- Safety
- Nutrition
- IV
- Intake and Output

Remember, each hospital selects its own codes. The codes used in the EPR at Pacific View Regional Hospital may be different from ones you have seen in your clinical rotations. Take some time to acquaint yourself with the codes. Within the Vital Signs category, click on any item in the left column (e.g., Pain: Characteristics). In the far-right column, you will see a list of code meanings for the possible findings and/or descriptors for that assessment area.

You will use the codes to record the data you collect as you work with patients. Click on the box in the last time column to the right of any item and wait for the code meanings applicable to that entry to appear. Select the appropriate code to describe your assessment findings and type it in the box. (*Note:* If no cursor appears within the box, click on the box again until the blue shading disappears and the blinking cursor appears.) Once the data are typed in this box, they are entered into the patient's record for this period of care only.

To leave the EPR, click on **Exit EPR** in the bottom right corner of the screen.

■ VISITING A PATIENT

From the Nurses' Station, click on the room number of the patient you wish to visit (in the tool bar at the bottom of your screen). Once you are inside the room, you will see a still photo of your patient in the top left corner. To verify that this is the correct patient, click on the **Check Armband** icon to the right of the photo. The patient's identification data will appear. If you click on **Check Allergies** (the next icon to the right), a list of the patient's allergies (if any) will replace the photo.

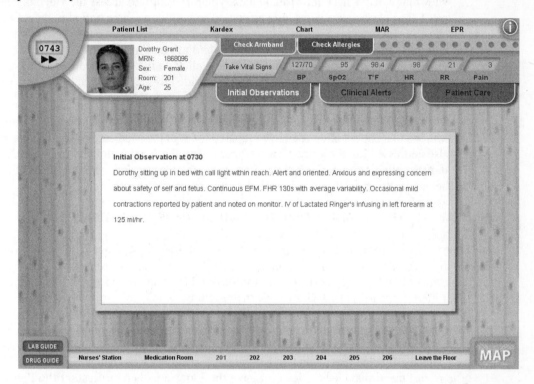

Also located in the patient's room are multiple icons you can use to assess the patient or the patient's medications. A virtual clock is provided in the upper left corner of the room to monitor your progress in real time. (*Note:* The fast-forward icon within the virtual clock will advance the time by 2-minute intervals when clicked.)

- The tool bar across the top of the screen allows you to check the **Patient List**, access the **EPR** to check or enter data, and view the patient's **Chart**, **MAR**, or **Kardex**.

- The **Take Vital Signs** icon allows you to measure the patient's up-to-the-minute blood pressure, oxygen saturation, temperature, heart rate, respiratory rate, and pain level.

- Each time you enter a patient's room, you are given an Initial Observation report to review (in the text box under the patient's photo). These notes are provided to give you a "look" at the patient as if you had just stepped into the room. You can also click on the **Initial Observations** icon to return to this box from other views within the patient's room. To the right of this icon is **Clinical Alerts**, a resource that allows you to make decisions about priority medication interventions based on emerging data collected in real time. Check this screen throughout your period of care to avoid missing critical information related to recently ordered or STAT medications.

- Clicking on **Patient Care** opens up three specific learning environments within the patient room: **Physical Assessment**, **Nurse-Client Interactions**, and **Medication Administration**.

- To perform a **Physical Assessment**, choose a body area (such as **Head & Neck**) from the column of yellow buttons. This activates a list of system subcategories for that body area (e.g., see **Sensory**, **Neurologic**, etc. in the green boxes). After you select the system you wish to evaluate, a brief description of the assessment findings will appear in a box to the right. A still photo provides a "snapshot" of how an assessment of this area might be done or what the finding might look like. For every body area, you can also click on **Equipment** on the right side of the screen.

- To the right of the Physical Assessment icon is **Nurse-Client Interactions**. Clicking on this icon will reveal the times and titles of any videos available for viewing. (*Note:* If the video you wish to see is not listed, this means you have not yet reached the correct virtual time to view that video. Check the virtual clock; you may return to access the video once its designated time has occurred—as long as you do so within the same period of care. Or you can click on the fast-forward icon within the virtual clock to advance the time by 2-minute intervals. You will then need to click again on **Patient Care** and **Nurse-Client Interactions** to refresh the screen.) To view a listed video, click on the white arrow to the right of the video title. Use the control buttons below the video to start, stop, pause, rewind, or fast-forward the action or to mute the sound.

- **Medication Administration** is the pathway that allows you to review and administer medications to a patient after you have prepared them in the Medication Room. This process is also addressed further in the *How to Prepare Medications* section below and in *Medications* in **A Detailed Tour**. For additional hands-on practice, see *Reducing Medication Errors* below **A Quick Tour** and **A Detailed Tour** in your resources.

■ HOW TO QUIT, CHANGE PATIENTS, OR CHANGE PERIODS OF CARE

How to Quit: From most screens, you may click the **Leave the Floor** icon on the bottom tool bar to the right of the patient room numbers. (*Note:* From some screens, you will first need to click an **Exit** button or **Return to Nurses' Station** before clicking **Leave the Floor**.) When the Floor Menu appears, click **Exit** to leave the program.

How to Change Patients or Periods of Care: To change patients, simply click on the new patient's room number. (You cannot receive a scorecard for a new patient, however, unless you have already selected that patient on the Patient List screen.) To change to a new period of care or to restart the virtual clock, click on **Leave the Floor** and then on **Restart the Program**.

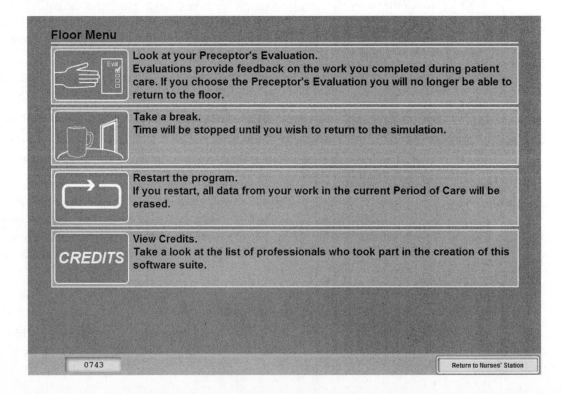

■ HOW TO PREPARE MEDICATIONS

From the Nurses' Station or the patient's room, you can access the Medication Room by clicking on the icon in the tool bar at the bottom of your screen to the left of the patient room numbers.

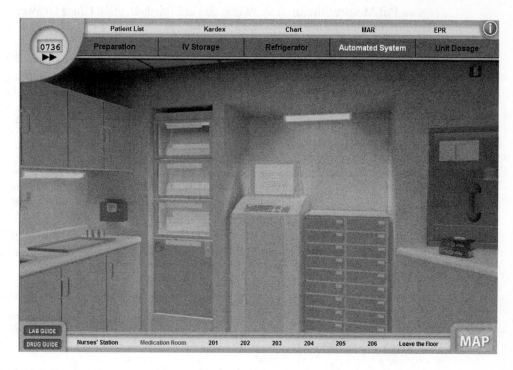

In the Medication Room you have access to the following (from left to right):

- A preparation area is located on the counter under the cabinets. To begin the medication preparation process, click on the tray on the counter or click on the **Preparation** icon at the top of the screen. The next screen leads you through a specific sequence (called the Preparation Wizard) to prepare medications one at a time for administration to a patient. However, no medication has been selected at this time. We will do this while working with a patient in **A Detailed Tour**. To exit this screen, click on **View Medication Room**.

- To the right of the cabinets (and above the refrigerator), IV storage bins are provided. Click on the bins themselves or on the **IV Storage** icon at the top of the screen. The bins are labeled **Microinfusion**, **Small Volume**, and **Large Volume**. Click on an individual bin to see a list of its contents. If you needed to prepare an IV medication at this time, you could click on the medication and its label would appear to the right under the patient's name. (*Note:* You can **Open** and **Close** any medication label by clicking the appropriate icon.) Next, you would click **Put Medication on Tray**. If you ever change your mind or decide that you have put the incorrect medication on the tray, you can reverse your actions by highlighting the medication on the tray and then clicking **Put Medication in Bin**. Click **Close Bin** in the right bottom corner to exit. **View Medication Room** brings you back to a full view of the entire room.

- A refrigerator is located under the IV storage bins to hold any medications that must be stored below room temperature. Click on the refrigerator door or on the **Refrigerator** icon at the top of the screen. Then click on the close-up view of the door to access the medications. When you are finished, click **Close Door** and then **View Medication Room**.

- To prepare controlled substances, click the **Automated System** icon at the top of the screen or click the computer monitor located to the right of the IV storage bins. A login screen will appear; your name and password are automatically filled in. Click **Login**. Select the patient for whom you wish to access medications; then select the correct medication drawer to open (they are stored alphabetically). Click **Open Drawer**, highlight the proper medication, and choose **Put Medication on Tray**. When you are finished, click **Close Drawer** and then **View Medication Room**.

- Next to the Automated System is a set of drawers identified by patient room number. To access these, click on the drawers or on the **Unit Dosage** icon at the top of the screen. This provides a close-up view of the drawers. To open a drawer, click on the room number of the patient you are working with. Next, click on the medication you would like to prepare for the patient, and a label will appear, listing the medication strength, units, and dosage per unit. To exit, click **Close Drawer**; then click **View Medication Room**.

At any time, you can learn about a medication you wish to prepare for a patient by clicking on the **Drug** icon in the bottom left corner of the medication room screen or by clicking the **Drug Guide** book on the counter to the right of the unit dosage drawers. The **Drug Guide** provides information about the medications commonly included in nursing drug handbooks. Nutritional supplements and maintenance intravenous fluid preparations are not included. Highlight a medication in the alphabetical list; relevant information about the drug will appear in the screen below. To exit, click **Return to Medication Room**.

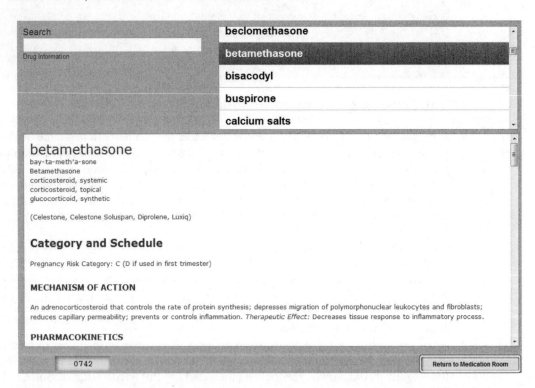

To access the MAR from the Medication Room and to review the medications ordered for a patient, click on the **MAR** icon located in the tool bar at the top of your screen and then click on the correct tab for your patient's room number. You may also click the **Review MAR** icon in the tool bar at the bottom of your screen from inside each medication storage area.

After you have chosen and prepared medications, go to the patient's room to administer them by clicking on the room number in the bottom tool bar. Inside the patient's room, click **Patient Care** and then **Medication Administration** and follow the proper administration sequence.

■ PRECEPTOR'S EVALUATIONS

When you have finished a session, click on **Leave the Floor** to go to the Floor Menu. At this point, you can click on the top icon (**Look at Your Preceptor's Evaluation**) to receive a scorecard that provides feedback on the work you completed during patient care.

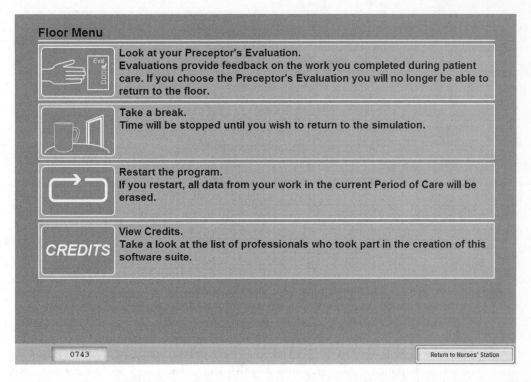

Evaluations are available for each patient you selected when you signed in for the current period of care. Click on the **Medication Scorecard** icon to see an example.

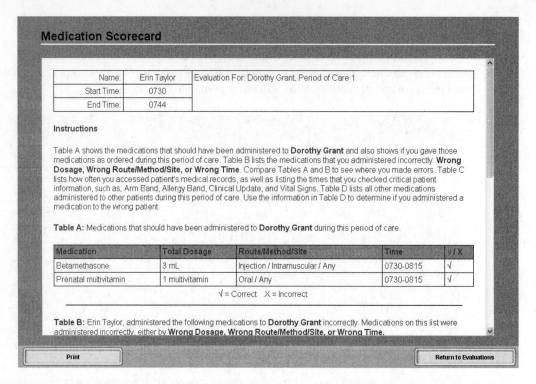

The scorecard compares the medications you administered to a patient during a period of care with what should have been administered. Table A lists the correct medications. Table B lists any medications that were administered incorrectly.

Remember, not every medication listed on the MAR should necessarily be given. For example, a patient might have an allergy to a drug that was ordered, or a medication might have been improperly transcribed to the MAR. Predetermined medication "errors" embedded within the program challenge you to exercise critical thinking skills and professional judgment when deciding to administer a medication, just as you would in a real hospital. Use all your available resources, such as the patient's chart and the MAR, to make your decision.

Table C lists the resources that were available to assist you in medication administration. It also documents whether and when you accessed these resources. For example, did you check the patient armband or perform a check of vital signs? If so, when?

You can click **Print** to get a copy of this report if needed. When you have finished reviewing the scorecard, click **Return to Evaluations** and then **Return to Menu**.

■ FLOOR MAP

To get a general sense of your location within the hospital, you can click on the **Map** icon found in the lower right corner of most of the screens in the *Virtual Clinical Excursions—Obstetrics* program. (*Note:* If you are following this quick tour step by step, you will need to **Restart the Program** from the Floor Menu, sign in again, and go to the Nurses' Station to access the map.) When you click the **Map** icon, a floor map appears, showing the layout of the floor you are currently on, as well as a directory of the patients and services on that floor. As you move your cursor over the directory list, the location of each room is highlighted on the map (and vice versa). The floor map can be accessed from the Nurses' Station, Medication Room, and each patient's room.

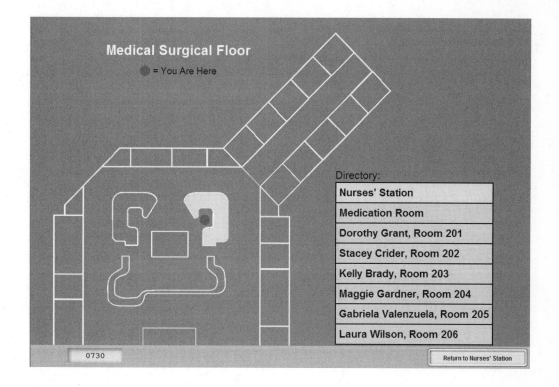

A DETAILED TOUR

If you wish to more thoroughly understand the capabilities of *Virtual Clinical Excursions—Obstetrics*, take a detailed tour by completing the following section. During this tour, we will work with a specific patient to introduce you to all the different components and learning opportunities available within the software.

■ WORKING WITH A PATIENT

Sign in for Period of Care 1 (0730-0815). From the Patient List, select Dorothy Grant in Room 201; however, do not go to the Nurses' Station yet.

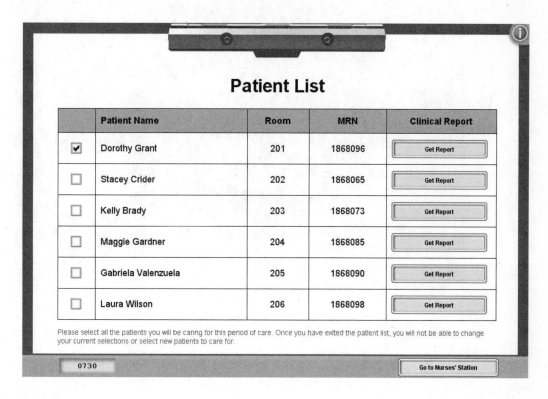

■ REPORT

In hospitals, when one shift ends and another begins, the outgoing nurse who attended a patient will give a verbal and sometimes a written summary of that patient's condition to the incoming nurse who will assume care for the patient. This summary is called a report and is an important source of data to provide an overview of a patient. Your first task is to get the clinical report on Dorothy Grant. To do this, click **Get Report** in the far right column in this patient's row. From a brief review of this summary, identify the problems and areas of concern that you will need to address for this patient.

When you have finished noting any areas of concern, click **Go to Nurses' Station**.

■ CHARTS

You can access Dorothy Grant's chart from the Nurses' Station or from the patient's room (201). From the Nurses' Station, click on the chart rack or on the **Chart** icon in the tool bar at the top of your screen. Next, click on the chart labeled **201** to open the medical record for Dorothy Grant. Click on the **Emergency Department** tab to view a record of why this patient was admitted.

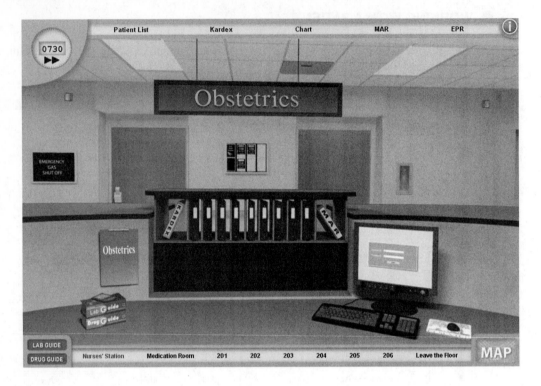

How many days has Dorothy Grant been in the hospital?

What tests were done upon her arrival in the Emergency Department and why?

What was the reason for her admission?

You should also click on **Diagnostic Reports** to learn what additional tests or procedures were performed and when. Finally, review the **Nursing Admission** and **History and Physical** to learn about the health history of this patient. When you are done reviewing the chart, click **Return to Nurses' Station**.

■ MEDICATIONS

Open the Medication Administration Record (MAR) by clicking on the **MAR** icon in the tool bar at the top of your screen. *Remember:* The MAR automatically opens to the first occupied room number on the floor—which is not necessarily your patient's room number! Since you need to access Dorothy Grant's MAR, click on tab **201** (her room number). Always make sure you are giving the *Right Drug to the Right Patient!*

Examine the list of medications ordered for Dorothy Grant. In the table below, list the medications that need to be given during this period of care (0730-0815). For each medication, note the dosage, route, and time to be given.

Time	Medication	Dosage	Route

Click on **Return to Nurses' Station**. Next, click on **201** on the bottom tool bar and then verify that you are indeed in Dorothy Grant's room. Select **Clinical Alerts** (the icon to the right of Initial Observations) to check for any emerging data that might affect your medication administration priorities. Next, go to the patient's chart (click on the **Chart** icon; then click on **201**). When the chart opens, select the **Physician's Orders** tab.

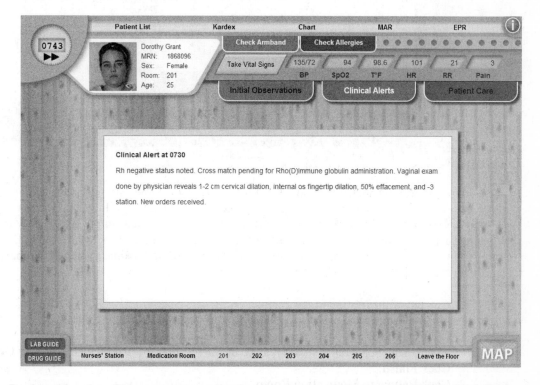

Review the orders. Have any new medications been ordered? Return to the MAR (click **Return to Room 201**; then click **MAR**). Verify that any new medications have been correctly transcribed to the MAR. Mistakes are sometimes made in the transcription process in the hospital setting, and it is sound practice to double-check any new order.

Are there any patient assessments you will need to perform before administering these medications? If so, return to Room 201 and click on **Patient Care** and then **Physical Assessment** to complete those assessments before proceeding.

Now click on the **Medication Room** icon in the tool bar at the bottom of your screen to locate and prepare the medications for Dorothy Grant.

In the Medication Room, you must access the medications for Dorothy Grant from the specific dispensing system in which each medication is stored. Locate each medication that needs to be given in this time period and click on **Put Medication on Tray** as appropriate. (*Hint:* Look in **Unit Dosage** drawer first.) When you are finished, click on **Close Drawer** and then on **View Medication Room**. Now click on the medication tray on the counter on the left side of the medication room screen to begin preparing the medications you have selected. (*Remember:* You can also click **Preparation** in the tool bar at the top of the screen.)

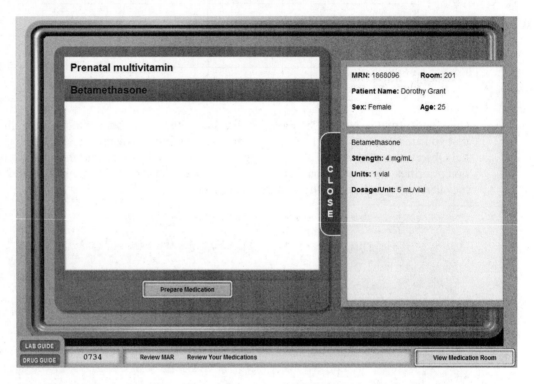

In the preparation area, you should see a list of the medications you put on the tray in the previous steps. Click on the first medication and then click **Prepare**. Follow the onscreen instructions of the Preparation Wizard, providing any data requested. As an example, let's follow the preparation process for betamethasone, one of the medications due to be administered to Dorothy Grant during this period of care. To begin, click on **Betamethasone**; then click **Prepare**. Now work through the Preparation Wizard sequence as detailed below:

> Amount of medication in the ampule: 5 mL.
> Enter the amount of medication you will draw up into a syringe: **3** mL.
> Click **Next**.
> Select the patient you wish to set aside the medication for: **Room 201, Dorothy Grant**.
> Click **Finish**.
> Click **Return to Medication Room**.

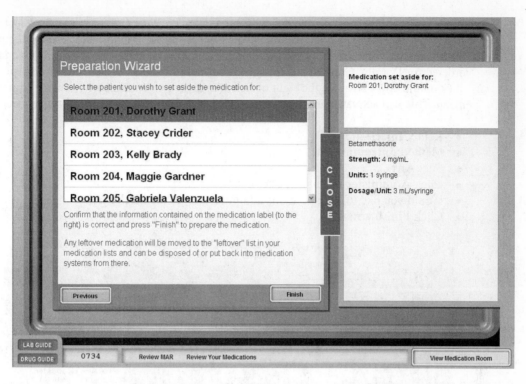

Follow this same basic process for the other medications due to be administered to Dorothy Grant during this period of care. (*Hint:* Look in **IV Storage** and **Automated System**.)

PREPARATION WIZARD EXCEPTIONS

- Some medications in *Virtual Clinical Excursions—Obstetrics* are prepared by the pharmacy (e.g., IV antibiotics) and taken to the patient room as a whole. This is common practice in most hospitals.
- Blood products are not administered by students through the *Virtual Clinical Excursions—Obstetrics* simulations since blood administration follows specific protocols not covered in this program.
- The *Virtual Clinical Excursions—Obstetrics* simulations do not allow for mixing more than one type of medication, such as regular and Lente insulins, in the same syringe. In the clinical setting, when multiple types of insulin are ordered for a patient, the regular insulin is drawn up first, followed by the longer-acting insulin. Insulin is always administered in a special unit-marked syringe.

Now return to Room 201 (click on **201** on the bottom tool bar) to administer Dorothy Grant's medications.

At any time during the medication administration process, you can perform a further review of systems, take vital signs, check information contained within the chart, or verify patient identity and allergies. Inside Dorothy Grant's room, click **Take Vital Signs**. (*Note:* These findings change over time to reflect the temporal changes you would find in a patient similar to Dorothy Grant.)

When you have gathered all the data you need, click on **Patient Care** and then select **Medication Administration**. Any medications you prepared in the previous steps should be listed on the left side of your screen. Let's continue the administration process with the betamethasone ordered for Dorothy Grant. Click to highlight **Betamethasone** in the list of medications. Next, click on the down arrow to the right of **Select** and choose **Administer** from the drop-down menu. This will activate the Administration Wizard. Complete the Wizard sequence as follows:

- Route: **Injection**
- Method: **Intramuscular**
- Site: **Any**
- Click **Administer to Patient** arrow.
- Would you like to document this administration in the MAR? **Yes**
- Click **Finish** arrow.

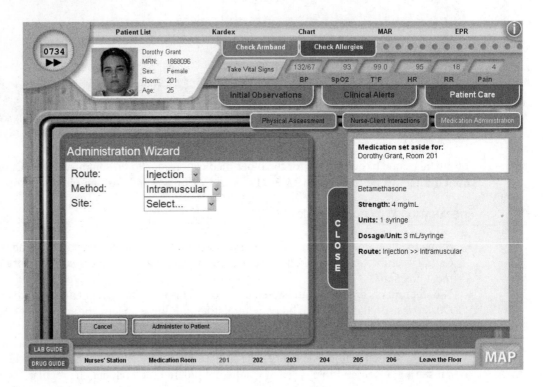

Your selections are recorded by a tracking system and evaluated on a Medication Scorecard stored under Preceptor's Evaluations. This scorecard can be viewed, printed, and given to your instructor. To access the Preceptor's Evaluations, click on **Leave the Floor**. When the Floor Menu appears, select **Look at Your Preceptor's Evaluation**. Then click on **Medication Scorecard** inside the box with Dorothy Grant's name (see example on the following page).

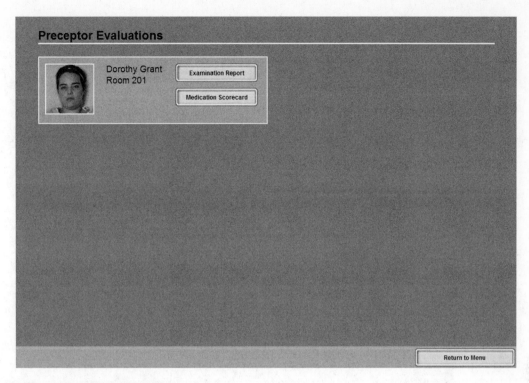

■ MEDICATION SCORECARD

- First, review Table A. Was betamethasone given correctly? Did you give the other medications as ordered?
- Table B shows you which (if any) medications you gave incorrectly.
- Table C addresses the resources used for Dorothy Grant. Did you access the patient's chart, MAR, EPR, or Kardex as needed to make safe medication administration decisions?
- Did you check the patient's armband to verify her identity? Did you check whether your patient had any known allergies to medications? Were vital signs taken?

When you have finished reviewing the scorecard, click **Return to Evaluations** and then **Return to Menu**.

■ **VITAL SIGNS**

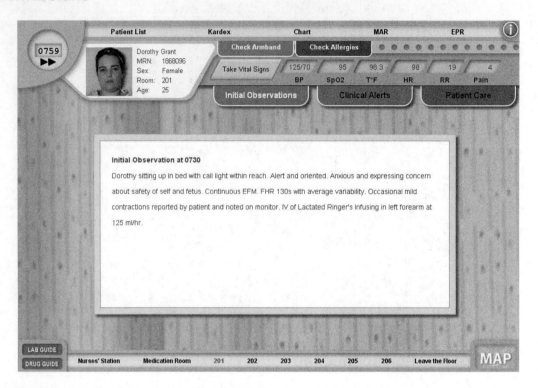

Vital signs, often considered the traditional "signs of life," include body temperature, heart rate, respiratory rate, blood pressure, oxygen saturation of the blood, and pain level.

Inside Dorothy Grant's room, click **Take Vital Signs**. (*Note:* If you are following this detailed tour step by step, you will need to **Restart the Program** from the Floor Menu, sign in again for Period of Care 1, and navigate to Room 201.) Collect vital signs for this patient and record them below. Note the time at which you collected each of these data. (*Remember:* You can take vital signs at any time. The data change over time to reflect the temporal changes you would find in a patient similar to Dorothy Grant.)

Vital Signs	Findings/Time
Blood pressure	
O$_2$ saturation	
Temperature	
Heart rate	
Respiratory rate	
Pain rating	

After you are done, click on the **EPR** icon located in the tool bar at the top of the screen. Your username and password are automatically provided. Click on **Login** to enter the EPR. To access Dorothy Grant's records, click on the down arrow next to Patient and choose her room number, **201**. Select **Vital Signs** as the category. Next, in the empty time column on the far right, record the vital signs data you just collected in the patient's room. If you need help with this process, refer to the Electronic Patient Record (EPR) section of the Quick Tour. Now compare these findings with the data you collected earlier for this patient's vital signs. Use these earlier findings to establish a baseline for each of the vital signs.

    a.   Are any of the data you collected significantly different from the baseline for a particular vital sign?

        Circle One: Yes   No

    b.   If "Yes," which data are different?

■ PHYSICAL ASSESSMENT

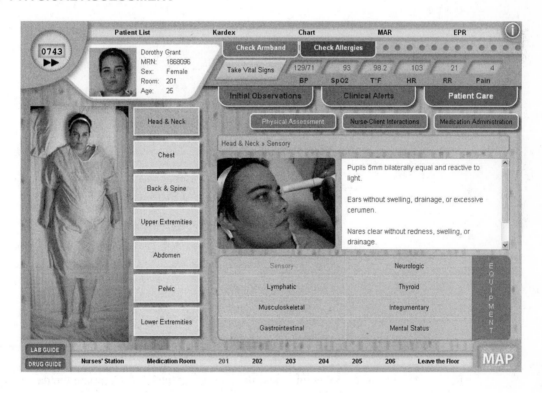

After you have finished examining the EPR for vital signs, click **Exit EPR** to return to Room 201. Click **Patient Care** and then **Physical Assessment**. Think about the information you received in the report at the beginning of this shift, as well as what you may have learned about this patient from the chart. Based on this, what area(s) of examination should you pay most attention to at this time? Is there any equipment you should be monitoring? Conduct a physical assessment of the body areas and systems that you consider priorities for Dorothy Grant. For example, select **Head & Neck**; then click on and assess **Sensory** and **Lymphatic**. Complete any other assessment(s) you think are necessary at this time. In the following table, record the data you collected during this examination.

Area of Examination	Findings
Head & Neck Sensory	
Head & Neck Lymphatic	

After you have finished collecting these data, return to the EPR. Compare the data that were already in the record with those you just collected.

    a. Are any of the data you collected significantly different from the baselines for this patient?

       Circle One: Yes   No

    b. If "Yes," which data are different?

■ NURSE-CLIENT INTERACTIONS

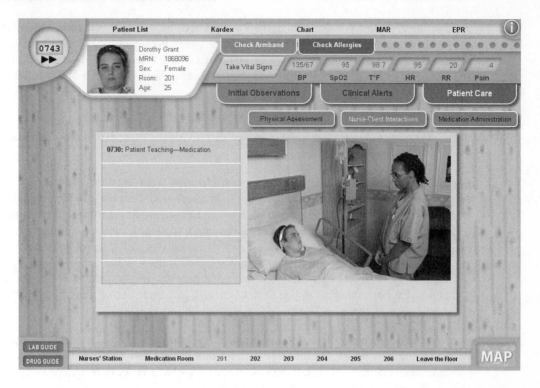

Click on **Patient Care** from inside Dorothy Grant's room (201). Now click on **Nurse-Client Interactions** to access a short video titled **Patient Teaching—Medication**, which is available for viewing at or after 0730 (based on the virtual clock in the upper left corner of your screen; see *Note* below). To begin the video, click on the white arrow next to its title. You will observe a nurse communicating with Dorothy Grant. There are many variations of nursing practice, some exemplifying "best" practice and some not. Note whether the nurse in this interaction displays professional behavior and compassionate care. Are her words congruent with what is going on with the patient? Does this interaction "feel right" to you? If not, how would you handle this situation differently? Explain.

Note: If the video you wish to view is not listed, this means you have not yet reached the correct virtual time to view that video. Check the virtual clock; you may return to access the video once its designated time has occurred—as long as you do so within the same period of care. Or you can click on the fast-forward icon within the virtual clock to advance the time by 2-minute intervals. You will then need to click again on **Patient Care** and **Nurse-Client Interactions** to refresh the screen.

At least one Nurse-Client Interactions video is available during each period of care. Viewing these videos can help you learn more about what is occurring with a patient at a certain time and also prompt you to discern between nurse communications that are ideal and those that need improvement. Compassionate care and the ability to communicate clearly are essential components of delivering quality nursing care, and it is during your clinical time that you will begin to refine these skills.

■ COLLECTING AND EVALUATING DATA

Each of the activities you perform in the Patient Care environment generates a significant amount of assessment data. Remember that after you collect data, you can record your findings in the EPR. You can also review the EPR, patient's chart, videos, and MAR at any time. You will get plenty of practice collecting and then evaluating data in context of the patient's course.

Now, here's an important question for you:

> Did the previous sequence of exercises provide the most efficient way to assess Dorothy Grant?

For example, you went to the patient's room to get vital signs, then back to the EPR to enter data and compare your findings with extant data. Next, you went back to the patient's room to do a physical examination, then again back to the EPR to enter and review data. If this back-and-forth process of data collection and recording seemed inefficient, remember the following:

- Plan all of your nursing activities to maximize efficiency, while at the same time optimizing the quality of patient care. (Think about what data you might need before performing certain tasks. For example, do you need to check a heart rate before administering a cardiac medication or check an IV site before starting an infusion?)

- You collect a tremendous amount of data when you work with a patient. Very few people can accurately remember all these data for more than a few minutes. Develop efficient assessment skills, and record data as soon as possible after collecting them.

- Assessment data are only the starting point for the nursing process.

Make a clear distinction between these first exercises and how you actually provide nursing care. These initial exercises were designed to involve you actively in the use of different software components. This workbook focuses on sensible practices for implementing the nursing process in ways that ensure the highest-quality care of patients.

Most important, remember that a human being changes through time, and that these changes include both the physical and psychosocial facets of a person as a living organism. Think about this for a moment. Some patients may change physically in a very short time (a patient with emerging myocardial infarction) or more slowly (a patient with a chronic illness). Patients' overall physical and psychosocial conditions may improve or deteriorate. They may have effective coping skills and familial support, or they may feel alone and full of despair. In fact, each individual is a complex mix of physical and psychosocial elements, and at least some of these elements usually change through time.

Thus it is crucial that you *DO NOT* think of the nursing process as a simple one-time, five-step procedure consisting of assessment, nursing diagnosis, planning, implementation, and evaluation. Rather, the nursing process should be utilized as a creative and systematic approach to delivering nursing care. Furthermore, because all living organisms are constantly changing, we must apply the nursing process over and over. Each time we follow the nursing process for an individual patient, we refine our understanding of that patient's physical and psychosocial conditions based on collection and analysis of many different types of data. *Virtual Clinical Excursions—Obstetrics* will help you develop both the creativity and the systematic approach needed to become a nurse who is equipped to deliver the highest-quality care to all patients.

REDUCING MEDICATION ERRORS

Earlier in the detailed tour, you learned the basic steps of medication preparation and administration. The following simulations will allow you to practice those skills further—with an increased emphasis on reducing medication errors by using the Medication Scorecard to evaluate your work.

Sign in to work on the Obstetrics Floor at Pacific View Regional Hospital for Period of Care 1. (*Note:* If you are already working with another patient or during another period of care, click on **Leave the Floor** and then **Restart the Program**; then sign in.)

From the Patient List, select Dorothy Grant. Then click on **Go to Nurses' Station**. Complete the following steps to prepare and administer medications to Dorothy Grant.

- Click on **Medication Room** on the tool bar at the bottom of your screen.

- Click on **MAR** and then on tab **201** to determine medications that have been ordered for Dorothy Grant. (*Note:* You may click on **Review MAR** at any time to verify the correct medication order. Always remember to check the patient name on the MAR to make sure you have the correct patient's record. You must click on the correct room number tab within the MAR.) Click on **Return to Medication Room** after reviewing the correct MAR.

- Click on **Unit Dosage** (or on the Unit Dosage cabinet); from the close-up view, click on drawer **201**.

- Select the medications you would like to administer. After each selection, click **Put Medication on Tray**. When you are finished selecting medications, click **Close Drawer** and then **View Medication Room**.

- Click **Automated System** (or on the Automated System unit itself). Click **Login**.

- On the next screen, specify the correct patient and drawer location.

- Select the medication you would like to administer and click **Put Medication on Tray**. Repeat this process if you wish to administer other medications from the Automated System.

- When you are finished, click **Close Drawer** and **View Medication Room**.

- From the Medication Room, click **Preparation** (or on the preparation tray).

- From the list of medications on your tray, highlight the correct medication to administer and click **Prepare**.

- This activates the Preparation Wizard. Supply any requested information; then click **Next**.

- Now select the correct patient to receive this medication and click **Finish**.

- Repeat the previous three steps until all medications that you want to administer are prepared.

- You can click on **Review Your Medications** and then on **Return to Medication Room** when ready. Once you are back in the Medication Room, go directly to Dorothy Grant's room by clicking on **201** at the bottom of the screen.

- Inside the patient's room, administer the medication, utilizing the six rights of medication administration. After you have collected the appropriate assessment data and are ready for administration, click **Patient Care** and then **Medication Administration**. Verify that the correct patient and medication(s) appear in the left-hand window. Highlight the first medication you wish to administer; then click the down arrow next to Select. From the drop-down menu, select **Administer** and complete the Administration Wizard by providing any information requested. When the Wizard stops asking for information, click **Administer to Patient**. Specify **Yes** when asked whether this administration should be recorded in the MAR. Finally, click **Finish**.

■ **SELF-EVALUATION**

Now let's see how you did during your medication administration!

• Click on **Leave the Floor** at the bottom of your screen. From the Floor Menu, select **Look at Your Preceptor's Evaluation**. Then click **Medication Scorecard**.

The following exercises will help you identify medication errors, investigate possible reasons for these errors, and reduce or prevent medication errors in the future.

1. Start by examining Table A. These are the medications you should have given to Dorothy Grant during this period of care. If each of the medications in Table A has a ✓ by it, then you made no errors. Congratulations!

If any medication has an X by it, then you made one or more medication errors.

Compare Tables A and B to determine which of the following types of errors you made: Wrong Dose, Wrong Route/Method/Site, or Wrong Time. Follow these steps:
   a. Find medications in Table A that were given incorrectly.
   b. Now see if those same medications are in Table B, which shows what you actually administered to Dorothy Grant.
   c. Comparing Tables A and B, match the Strength, Dose, Route/Method/Site, and Time for each medication you administered incorrectly.
   d. Then, using the form below, list the medications given incorrectly and mark the errors you made for each medication.

Medication	Strength	Dosage	Route	Method	Site	Time
	❑	❑	❑	❑	❑	❑
	❑	❑	❑	❑	❑	❑
	❑	❑	❑	❑	❑	❑
	❑	❑	❑	❑	❑	❑

2. To help you reduce future medication errors, consider the following list of possible reasons for errors.

• Did not check drug against MAR for correct medication, correct dose, correct patient, correct route, correct time, correct documentation.
• Did not check drug dose against MAR three times.
• Did not open the unit dose package in the patient's room.
• Did not correctly identify the patient using two identifiers.
• Did not administer the drug on time.
• Did not verify patient allergies.
• Did not check the patient's current condition or vital sign parameters.
• Did not consider why the patient would be receiving this drug.
• Did not question why the drug was in the patient's drawer.
• Did not check the physician's order and/or check with the pharmacist when there was a question about the drug or dose.
• Did not verify that no adverse effects had occurred from a previous dose.

Based on the list of possibilities you just reviewed, determine how you made each error and record the reason in the form below:

Medication	Reason for Error

3. Look again at Table B. Are there medications listed that are not in Table A? If so, you gave a medication to Dorothy Grant that she should not have received. Complete the following exercises to help you understand how such an error might have been made.

    a. Perhaps you gave a medication that was on Dorothy Grant's MAR for this period of care, without recognizing that a change had occurred in the patient's condition, which should have caused you to reconsider. Review patient records as necessary and complete the following form:

Medication	Possible Reasons Not to Give This Medication

    b. Another possibility is that you gave Dorothy Grant a medication that should have been given at a different time. Check her MAR and complete the form below to determine whether you made a Wrong Time error:

Medication	Given to Dorothy Grant at What Time	Should Have Been Given at What Time

c. Maybe you gave another patient's medication to Dorothy Grant. In this case, you made a Wrong Patient error. Check the MARs of other patients and use the form below to determine whether you made this type of error:

Medication	Given to Dorothy Grant	Should Have Been Given to

4. The Medication Scorecard provides some other interesting sources of information. For example, if there is a medication selected for Dorothy Grant but it was not given to her, there will be an X by that medication in Table A, but it will not appear in Table B. In that case, you might have given this medication to some other patient, which is another type of Wrong Patient error. To investigate further, look at Table D, which lists the medications you gave to other patients. See whether you can find any medications ordered for Dorothy Grant that were given to another patient by mistake. However, before you make any decisions, be sure to cross-check the MAR for other patients because the same medication may have been ordered for multiple patients. Use the following form to record your findings:

Medication	Should Have Been Given to Dorothy Grant	Given by Mistake to

5. Now take some time to review the medication exercises you just completed. Use the form below to create an overall analysis of what you have learned. Once again, record each of the medication errors you made, including the type of each error. Then, for each error you made, indicate specifically what you would do differently to prevent this type of error from occurring again.

Medication	Type of Error	Error Prevention Tactic

Submit this form to your instructor if required as a graded assignment, or simply use these exercises to improve your understanding of medication errors and how to reduce them.

Name: _____   Date: _____

LESSON **1**

Community Care:
The Family and Culture

Reading Assignment: Community Care: The Family and Culture (Chapter 2)

Patients: Dorothy Grant, Room 201
Stacey Crider, Room 202
Kelly Brady, Room 203
Maggie Gardner, Room 204
Gabriela Valenzuela, Room 205
Laura Wilson, Room 206

Goal: To demonstrate an understanding of how the family, community, and culture affect the pregnant woman.

Objectives:

- Discuss the various types of families, communities, and cultures represented by each of the patients.
- Assess and plan care for a patient from a specific culture.
- Explore how your background influences the care that you give to patients who have differing experiences in regard to community, family, or culture.

Exercise 1

Virtual Hospital Activity

15 minutes

Review Chapter 2 in your textbook and complete the following exercise regarding family types.

Read question 1 before starting this period of care. Fill in the table as you review each patient's chart.

- Sign in to work at Pacific View Regional Hospital for Period of Care 1. (*Note*: If you are already in the virtual hospital from a previous exercise, click on **Leave the Floor** and then on **Restart the Program** to get to the sign-in window.)

- From the Patient List, select all six patients.
- Click on **Go to Nurses' Station** and then on **Chart**.
- Click on **201** (Dorothy Grant's chart) to begin.
- Click on the **Admissions** tab and find the patient's marital status.
- Click on the **History and Physical** tab and review the Family History section.
- Once you have completed the column for Dorothy Grant in the table below, click on **Return to Nurses' Station**.
- Click on **Chart** and then on **202** (Stacey Crider's chart). Repeat this sequence until you have completed question 1.

1. Under each patient's name in the table below, place an X next to each description that applies to the patient's type of family.

	Dorothy Grant	Stacey Crider	Kelly Brady	Maggie Gardner	Gabriela Valenzuela	Laura Wilson
Nuclear						
Marriage-blended						
Extended						
Single-parent						
Multigenerational						

2. Using what you learned in your chart review combined with the information in your textbook, describe the type of family that Gabriela Valenzuela has.

3. Based on the information provided in your textbook, what type of family do you have? Describe how your family fits the description of the family type that you have chosen.

Exercise 2

Virtual Hospital Activity

15 minutes

Just as there are different types of families, there are also various populations of women within every community.

Read question 1 before starting this period of care. Fill in the table as you review each patient's chart.

- Sign in to work at Pacific View Regional Hospital for Period of Care 1. (*Note*: If you are already in the virtual hospital from a previous exercise, click on **Leave the Floor** and then on **Restart the Program** to get to the sign-in window.)
- From the Patient List, select all six patients.
- Click on **Go to Nurses' Station** and then on **Chart**.
- Click on **201** (Dorothy Grant's chart) to begin.
- Click on the **Nursing Admissions** tab. (*Hint*: The first four pages of this section will provide information regarding patient population.)
- Click on **History and Physical** and gather additional information needed to complete the table below.
- Once you have completed Dorothy Grant's column in question 1, click on **Return to Nurses' Station**.
- Click on **Chart** and then on **202** (Stacey Crider's chart). Repeat the above steps for each patient.

1. Under each patient's name in the table below, place an X next to each description that applies.

	Dorothy Grant	Stacey Crider	Kelly Brady	Maggie Gardner	Gabriela Valenzuela	Laura Wilson
Adolescent						
Minority						
Older						
Incarcerated						
Migrant						
Homeless						
Immigrant						

2. Laura Wilson is a member of one of the most medically underserved groups. What are two lifestyle choices she has made that represent high risk behaviors common in this group?

3. Dorothy Grant could be classified as homeless. What are two health problems frequently seen in homeless women?

4. Older pregnant women, such as Maggie Gardner, are less likely to use _____ services,

   leading to _____.

5. Minority women with underlying health conditions have an increased risk for

   _____ for _____ and

   _____.

6. What has your experience been in caring for patients with a similar set of circumstances?

7. Based on the information found in the textbook, will you change the way you care for these patients in the future? If so, how? In your community, what resources are available for women who are affected by the issues discussed in this exercise?

Exercise 3

Virtual Hospital Activity

20 minutes

- Sign in to work at Pacific View Regional Hospital for Period of Care 1. (*Note*: If you are already in the virtual hospital from a previous exercise, click on **Leave the Floor** and then on **Restart the Program** to get to the sign-in window.)
- From the Patient List, select Stacey Crider (Room 202) and Maggie Gardner (Room 204).
- Click on **Go to Nurses' Station**.
- Click on **Chart** and then on **202**.
- Click on the **Nursing Admission** tab.
- Review Stacey Crider's Nursing Admission. (*Hint*: See the Role Relationships section.)

1. Identify a nursing diagnosis that would be appropriate for Stacey Crider and her family.

- Click on **Return to Nurses' Station**.
- Click on **Chart** and then on **204**.
- Click on the **Nursing Admission** tab.
- Review Maggie Gardner's Nursing Admission. (*Hint*: See the Health Promotion section.)

2. What alternative therapy/complementary therapy does Maggie Gardner use to relieve stomach trouble?

3. According to Table 2-2 in the textbook, what are some cultural practices during pregnancy that are common in Maggie Gardner's cultural group?

Maggie Gardner and her husband are very religious. According to the textbook, most members of the African-American culture have strong feelings about family, community, and religion. With this information in mind, complete the following activity and questions.

- Click on **Return to Nurses' Station**.
- Click on **204** at the bottom of the screen.
- Click on **Patient Care** and then on **Nurse-Client Interactions**.

- Select and view the video titled **0730: Communicating Empathy**. (*Note:* Check the virtual clock to see whether enough time has elapsed. You can use the fast-forward feature to advance the time by 2-minute intervals if the video is not yet available. Then click again on **Patient Care** and **Nurse-Client Interactions** to refresh the screen.)

4. What does Maggie Gardner's husband verbalize during this interaction that would correlate with the African-American population's deep sense of religion?

5. Based on interactions with patients in the hospital where you have worked, describe your experience(s) with caring for someone of a different culture. What, if any, ideas did you encounter that differed from your own? What barriers did you encounter while providing care?

6. How comfortable are you with caring for patients from a different culture? Do you find yourself feeling judgmental or attempting to change others? What can you do to learn more about other cultures?

7. What resources are available at your hospital or within your community to enhance your ability to care for a culturally diverse population?

To further explore Jim and Maggie Gardner's spiritual perspective of the event at hand, return to the patient's chart.

- Click on **Chart** and then on **204**.
- Click on the **Consultations** tab.
- Review the Pastoral Care Spiritual Assessment and the Pastoral Consultation. (*Hint:* Be sure to scroll down to read all the pages in this section.)

8. What does Maggie Gardner "blame" her miscarriages on?

9. Based on your review, what is Maggie Gardner's perception of God?

10. Based on your review of Maggie Gardner's chart during this exercise, what is one underlying theme that you see in the Consultations, Nursing Admission, and History and Physical in regard to religion and this patient's perception of her situation?

LESSON **2**

Violence Against Women

Reading Assignment: Violence Against Women (Chapter 5)

Patient: Dorothy Grant, Room 201

Goal: To identify patients at risk for intimate partner violence (IPV), interventions to assist those at risk, and ways to educate and empower those individuals toward healthy relationships.

Objectives:

- Discuss the statistics related to IPV.
- List characteristics of individuals involved in IPV.
- Explore the myths and facts regarding IPV.
- Identify the nurse's role in regard to the battered woman or those affected by IPV.

Exercise 1

Writing Activity

10 minutes

1. Historically, women have often been treated inhumanely. This continues even today. Based on information from the textbook, indicate whether each of the following statements is true or false.

    a. _____   In ancient Roman times, women were provided fair and equal treatment in relation to acts of adultery and public drunkenness.

    b. _____   Sex trafficking victims may experience Stockholm Syndrome, in which victims become attached to their enslavers.

    c. _____   Until the nineteenth century, abuse of one's wife was legal in the United States.

    d. _____   Mental illness can be blamed for the majority of violent acts against women.

    e. _____   Children who are abused are more likely to abuse as adults than are children who have never been abused.

2. Abused women, regardless of socioeconomic level, are _____ _____.

3. A student nurse is reviewing information about IPV. Which of the following statements indicates an adequate understanding of the impact of culture on this phenomena?
    a. "African-American women are less likely to be victims of IPV."
    b. "The occurrence of IPV is relatively low in Native American women."
    c. "Native Alaskan women have the highest rate of IPV."
    d. "Hispanic women have the lowest rate of IPV."

4. Which of the following characteristics are often seen in a batterer? Select all that apply.

    _____ High self-esteem

    _____ Arrogance

    _____ Short temper

    _____ Inability to empathize with others

    _____ History of family violence during childhood

Exercise 2

Virtual Hospital Activity

45 minutes

- Sign in to work at Pacific View Regional Hospital for Period of Care 1. (*Note*: If you are already in the virtual hospital from a previous exercise, click on **Leave the Floor** and then on **Restart the Program** to get to the sign-in window.)
- From the Patient List, select Dorothy Grant (Room 201).
- Click on **Go to Nurses' Station**.
- Click on **Chart** and then on **201**.
- Click on the **Nursing Admission** tab.

In addition to reading about Dorothy Grant's perspective on her current situation, review the characteristics of battered women found in the textbook.

1. What is the reality of Dorothy Grant's situation? How does that correlate with the textbook reading?

- Still in Dorothy Grant's chart, click on and review the **History and Physical** and **Nursing Admission**.

2. For each characteristic of battered women listed below and on the next page, supply correlating data from Dorothy Grant's chart as applicable. Base your answers on what you have learned about the patient so far in your chart review. (*Note:* You will return to this list to add follow-up findings after viewing the 0810 video interaction between Dorothy Grant and the nurse.)

Financially dependent

Few resources/support systems

Fewer problem-solving skills

Social isolation

Blame themselves for what has taken place

State that they are not "good enough"

Bonding occurs out of fear and helplessness

Low self-esteem

History of domestic violence in their family

Strong nurturing, yielding personality

Tolerate control from others easily

Experience deliberate/repeated physical or sexual assault

- Click on **Return to Nurses' Station**.
- Click on **201** at the bottom of the screen.
- Click on **Patient Care** and then on **Nurse-Client Interactions**. (*Note:* Take notes as you watch the following video.)
- Select and view the video titled **0810: Monitoring/Patient Support**. (*Note:* Check the virtual clock to see whether enough time has elapsed. You can use the fast-forward feature to advance the time by 2-minute intervals if the video is not yet available. Then click again on **Patient Care** and **Nurse-Client Interactions** to refresh the screen.)

3. What does Dorothy Grant say that she should do in order to help prevent the violence?

4. What are the patient's concerns at the moment?

5. Return to question 2 and review your answers, keeping in mind what you have learned through the 0810 nurse-client interaction. Would you change any of your answers based on this observation? If so, what would you add or change?

Exercise 3

Virtual Hospital Activity

10 minutes

- Sign in to work at Pacific View Regional Hospital for Period of Care 3. (*Note:* If you are already in the virtual hospital from a previous exercise, click on **Leave the Floor** and then on **Restart the Program** to get to the sign-in window.)
- From the Patient List, select Dorothy Grant (Room 201).
- Click on **Go to Nurses' Station**.
- Click on **Chart** and then on **201**.
- Click on **Consultations** and review the Psychiatric Consult and the Social Work Consult.

Review the information regarding the myths and facts about IPV in the textbook. Based on that information and your review of Dorothy Grant's chart, answer the following questions.

1. Dorothy Grant stays in the relationship because of _____ and

   _____.

2. The nurse caring for Dorothy Grant recognizes that the percentage of women who are battered during pregnancy is:
   a. 1% to 5%.
   b. 4% to 8%.
   c. 5% to 9%.
   d. 8% to 12%.

3. Based on the information provided, in what phase of the abuse cycle is Dorothy Grant?

4. According to the consults, Dorothy Grant has several options. What are some of the options that the social worker and psychiatric health care provider can offer her or assist her with?

5. Pregnant adolescents have been found to be at very high risk for abuse during which period?
   a During the 1st trimester
   b. During the 2nd trimester
   c. During the 3rd trimester
   d. During the early postpartum period

6. Indicate whether each of the following statements is true or false.

   a. _____ Battering often escalates or begins during pregnancy.

   b. _____ Dorothy Grant's husband blames her for the pregnancy.

   c. _____ Dorothy Grant stays in the relationship because she likes to be beaten and deliberately provokes the attacks on occasion.

Exercise 4

Virtual Hospital Activity

10 minutes

- Sign in to work at Pacific View Regional Hospital for Period of Care 4. (*Note*: If you are already in the virtual hospital from a previous exercise, click on **Leave the Floor** and then on **Restart the Program** to get to the sign-in window.)
- From the Nurses' Station, click on **Kardex** and then on tab **201** to review Dorothy Grant's record. (*Remember:* You are not able to visit patients or administer medications during Period of Care 4. You are able to review patient records only.)

1. What action was initiated on Wednesday to protect Dorothy Grant from her husband?

2. What care plan diagnoses are appropriate for this patient's current life situation?

3. What other disciplines have been contacted or consulted that will ensure continuity of care for Dorothy Grant related to her abuse?

4. As a nurse caring for Dorothy Grant, what is your responsibility for reporting IPV?

5. When providing care to Dorothy Grant, a nurse must recognize which of the following complications as being related to violence during pregnancy? Select all that apply.

_____ Elevated weight gain

_____ Depression

_____ Suicide

_____ Substance abuse

6. When caring for Dorothy Grant, a nurse may implement the ABCDES tool. List appropriate interventions for Dorothy Grant using the ABCDES tool.

ABCDES	Intervention
A	
B	
C	
D	
E	
S	

7. What resources are available in your area for women who are experiencing IPV?

Reproductive System Concerns, Contraception, and Infertility

Reading Assignment: Reproductive System Concerns (Chapter 6)
Contraception and Abortion (Chapter 8)
Infertility (Chapter 9)

Patients: Stacey Crider, Room 202
Kelly Brady, Room 203
Maggie Gardner, Room 204
Gabriela Valenzuela, Room 205
Laura Wilson, Room 206

Goal: To demonstrate an understanding of reproductive system concerns, contraception options, and infertility.

Objectives:

- Identify potential reproductive issues.
- Differentiate between the various types of available contraception.
- Identify various methods of testing and treatment options for couples experiencing infertility.

Exercise 1

Virtual Hospital Activity

15 minutes

Review Chapter 6 in your textbook to answer the following questions.

1. What is a normal length for a menstrual cycle?

2. Menstruation is most irregular at the extremes of the reproductive years, including

_____ and _____.

3. When diagnosing an individual with amenorrhea, which of the following criteria are needed?
   a. A 6- to 12-month absence of menses after a period of menstruation
   b. Spotty menses in the absence of ovulation
   c. Absence of menses by age 18, regardless of the presence of normal growth and development
   d. Absence of both menarche and secondary sexual characteristics by age 14 years
   e. The occurrence of pain with menstruation

- Sign in to work at Pacific View Regional Hospital for Period of Care 1. (*Note*: If you are already in the virtual hospital from a previous exercise, click on **Leave the Floor** and then on **Restart the Program** to get to the sign-in window.)
- From the Patient List, select Stacey Crider (Room 202).
- Click on **Go to Nurses' Station**.
- Click on **Chart** and then on **202**.
- Click on **History and Physical**.
- Review the patient's gynecologic history.

4. Does Stacey Crider meet the textbook's criteria for amenorrhea?

5. What is her history?

6. List three things that can cause amenorrhea.

Exercise 2

Virtual Hospital Activity

20 minutes

Review Chapter 8 in your textbook to answer the following questions.

1. A nurse is assessing a patient's understanding regarding contraceptive methods. Which of the following responses indicates a lack of understanding? Select all that apply.

   _____ "To ensure protection, I should simultaneously use a male and female condom."

   _____ "The risk for breast cancer is increased with the use of oral contraceptives."

   _____ "Natural skin condoms may offer slightly more protection against infections than latex condoms."

_____ "When using a diaphragm with spermicide, the risk for pregnancy is less than 20%."

_____ "Toxic shock is a potential complication associated with the use of an intrauterine device (IUD)."

2. To ensure that informed consent has been provided to an individual concerning contraception, what should be reviewed?

3. _____ methods of contraception may provide some degree of protection from STIs.

- Sign in to work at Pacific View Regional Hospital for Period of Care 1. (*Note*: If you are already in the virtual hospital from a previous exercise, click on **Leave the Floor** and then on **Restart the Program** to get to the sign-in window.)
- From the Patient List, select Kelly Brady (Room 203), Gabriela Valenzuela (Room 205), and Laura Wilson (Room 206).
- Click on **Go to Nurses' Station**.
- Click on **Chart** and then on **203** for Kelly Brady's chart.
- Click on and review the **History and Physical**.
- Click on **Return to Nurses' Station** and repeat the previous two steps for Gabriela Valenzuela (205) and Laura Wilson (206).

4. Based on your review of the patients' charts, list the birth control method that each woman was using before her current pregnancy.

Kelly Brady

Gabriela Valenzuela

Laura Wilson

5. Gabriela Valenzuela is Catholic. Which method of contraception would be appropriate for the nurse to discuss with her?

6. During which of the following times is a woman considered to be the *most* fertile?
   a. 5 days after menstruation ceases
   b. 4 days before ovulation
   c. During menstruation
   d. 2 days following ovulation

7. Which of the following characteristics of cervical mucus is traditionally associated with increased levels of fertility?
   a. Thick, dense cervical mucus
   b. Clear, watery cervical mucus
   c. Cloudy, sticky cervical mucus
   d. Scant, cloudy cervical mucus

8. On what factor does the family planning method rely?

9. Laura Wilson is HIV-positive. What is the most appropriate form of birth control for her? Why?

10. _____ Nonoxynol-9, the active ingredient in spermicides, may be associated with an increase in the risk for contracting HIV. (True/False)

Exercise 3

Virtual Hospital Activity

30 minutes

Review Chapter 9 in your textbook.

1. _____% of the reproductive age population has a problem with infertility.

2. At the age of _____ the incidence of infertility in women increases.

Maggie Gardner is 41 years old. Let's consider some of the options she had while attempting to get pregnant.

3. List two factors that affect female fertility.

4. List two factors that affect male fertility.

LESSON 3—REPRODUCTIVE SYSTEM CONCERNS, CONTRACEPTION, AND INFERTILITY   57

- Sign in to work at Pacific View Regional Hospital for Period of Care 1. (*Note*: If you are already in the virtual hospital from a previous exercise, click on **Leave the Floor** and then on **Restart the Program** to get to the sign-in window.)
- From the Patient List, select Maggie Gardner (Room 204).
- Click on **Go to Nurses' Station**.
- Click on **Chart** and then on **204**.
- Review the **History and Physical**.

5. Maggie Gardner was married _____ years before conceiving the first time.

6. Based on the textbook reading, which of the following types of infertility would Maggie Gardner have been diagnosed with if she had chosen to get treatment after a year of attempting to get pregnant?
   a. Primary infertility
   b. Secondary infertility

7. List four tests that can be completed on a female patient to determine the causes of infertility.

8. List two tests that can be completed on a male patient to determine the causes of infertility.

9. A nurse is discussing the use of home-based ovulation predictor kits with a patient. The nurse correctly explains that the kit is used to detect an increase of which of the following in the woman's urine?
   a. Estrogen
   b. Follicle-stimulating hormone (FSH)
   c. Luteinizing hormone
   d. Progesterone

10. What methods are available to assist the infertile couple in conceiving?

11. What methods did Maggie Gardner and her husband use to assist in getting pregnant?

Copyright © 2015 by Mosby, an imprint of Elsevier Inc. All rights reserved.

Sexually Transmitted and Other Infections

Reading Assignment: Sexually Transmitted and Other Infections (Chapter 7)

Patients: Stacey Crider, Room 202
Gabriela Valenzuela, Room 205
Laura Wilson, Room 206

Goal: To demonstrate an understanding of the identification and management of selected sexually transmitted and other infections in pregnant women.

Objectives:

- Assess and plan care for a pregnant woman with bacterial vaginosis.
- Explain the importance of prophylactic group B streptococcus (GBS) treatment.
- Identify risk factors for acquiring human immunodeficiency virus (HIV).
- Prioritize information to be included in patient teaching related to HIV.

Exercise 1

Virtual Hospital Activity

15 minutes

- Sign in to work at Pacific View Regional Hospital for Period of Care 1. (*Note*: If you are already in the virtual hospital from a previous exercise, click on **Leave the Floor** and then on **Restart the Program** to get to the sign-in window.)
- From the Patient List, select Stacey Crider (Room 202).
- Click on **Go to Nurses' Station**.
- Click on **Chart** and then on **202**.
- Click on **History and Physical**.

1. Stacey Crider has been diagnosed with bacterial vaginosis. Which of the following characteristics is most consistent with this disorder?
   a. Foamy, yellow discharge
   b. Thick, white curd-like discharge
   c. Thin, grey-white discharge
   d. Green, watery discharge

2. How is bacterial vaginosis diagnosed?

3. Which of the following medications may be used to treat bacterial vaginosis during pregnancy?
   a. Metronidazole
   b. Diflucan
   c. Amoxicillin
   d. Acyclovir

- Now click on **Physician's Orders** in the chart.
- Scroll down to the admitting physician's orders on Tuesday at 0630.

4. _____, _____, and _____ are terms formerly used to refer to bacterial vaginosis.

5. What are Stacey Crider's admission diagnoses?

6. Explain how Stacey Crider's admission diagnoses are likely to be interrelated.

7. Which medication did Stacey Crider's physician order to treat her bacterial vaginosis?

8. _____ It is not necessary to treat Stacey Crider's partner for bacterial vaginosis. (True/False)

9. Assume that Stacey Crider is discharged home on day 4 of the prescribed treatment of the medication you identified in question 6. What specific information about this medication should be included as part of her discharge instructions?

Exercise 2

Virtual Hospital Activity

10 minutes

- Sign in to work at Pacific View Regional Hospital for Period of Care 1. (*Note*: If you are already in the virtual hospital from a previous exercise, click on **Leave the Floor** and then on **Restart the Program** to get to the sign-in window.)
- From the Patient List, select Gabriela Valenzuela (Room 205).
- Click on **Go to Nurses' Station**.
- Click on **Chart** and then on **205**.
- Click on **History and Physical** and scroll to the plan at the end of this document.

1. What is the medical plan of care for Gabriela Valenzuela?

2. Is Gabriela Valenzuela known to be positive for GBS?

3. According to the textbook, list the risk factors for neonatal GBS infection. Which risk factor applies to Gabriela Valenzuela?

4. Since pregnant women with GBS in the vagina are almost always asymptomatic, why does Gabriela Valenzuela need to be treated for this organism?

• Click on **Physician's Orders** and review the orders for Tuesday at 2100.

5. What medication/dosage/frequency will Gabriela Valenzuela receive for GBS prophylaxis?

6. How does this order compare with the treatment regimen recommended in your textbook?

Exercise 3

Virtual Hospital Activity

15 minutes

• Sign in to work at Pacific View Regional Hospital for Period of Care 1. (*Note*: If you are already in the virtual hospital from a previous exercise, click on **Leave the Floor** and then on **Restart the Program** to get to the sign-in window.)
• From the Patient List, select Laura Wilson (Room 206).
• Click on **Go to Nurses' Station**.
• Click on **Chart** and then on **206**.
• Click on **Nursing Admission**.

1. What factors identified on Laura Wilson's Nursing Admission form increase her risk for acquiring a sexually transmitted infection (STI)?

2. List specific risk factors for acquiring HIV. Underline the risk factors that are present in Laura Wilson's history.

3. What did the admitting nurse document about Laura Wilson's knowledge and acceptance of her HIV diagnosis?

- Click on **Return to Nurses' Station** and then on **206** at the bottom of the screen.
- Click on **Patient Care** and then on **Nurse-Client Interactions**.
- Select and view the video titled **0800: Teaching—HIV in Pregnancy**. (*Note:* Check the virtual clock to see whether enough time has elapsed. You can use the fast-forward feature to advance the time by 2-minute intervals if the video is not yet available. Then click again on **Patient Care** and **Nurse-Client Interactions** to refresh the screen.)

4. Does Laura Wilson appear to be fully aware of the implications of HIV? State the rationale for your answer.

5. What coping mechanism is Laura Wilson exhibiting in the video interaction?

- Click on **Chart** and then on **206**.
- Click on **Nursing Admission**.

6. Laura Wilson needs education on each of the topics listed below. Which topic would you choose to teach her about at this time?
   a. Safer sex
   b. Medication side effects and importance of compliance
   c. Need for medical follow-up and medication for the baby
   d. Impact of HIV on birth plans

7. Give a rationale for your answer to question 6.

LESSON 5
==

Assessment of Risk Factors in Pregnancy, Including Maternal and Fetal Nutrition

Reading Assignment: Maternal and Fetal Nutrition (Chapter 14)
Assessment for Risk Factors (Chapter 26)
Medical-Surgical Problems (Chapter 30)

Patients: Kelly Brady, Room 203
Maggie Gardner, Room 204
Laura Wilson, Room 206

Goal: To demonstrate an understanding of assessment for risk factors in pregnancy, including maternal and fetal nutritional aspects.

Objectives:

- Identify appropriate interventions for maintaining appropriate maternal and fetal nutrition.
- Differentiate between the various types of assessment techniques that can be used with both low and high risk pregnancy patients.
- Identify various methods of testing that can be used in high risk pregnancies.

Exercise 1

Virtual Hospital Activity

15 minutes

- Sign in to work at Pacific View Regional Hospital for Period of Care 1. (*Note*: If you are already in the virtual hospital from a previous exercise, click on **Leave the Floor** and then on **Restart the Program** to get to the sign-in window.)
- From the Patient List, select Maggie Gardner (Room 204).
- Click on **Go to Nurses' Station**.
- Click on **Chart** and then on **204**.
- Click on **Laboratory Reports**.
- Click on **History and Physical**.

Review Chapter 15 and Chapter 30 in your textbook.

1. What were Maggie Gardner's hemoglobin and hematocrit levels on admission?

2. Which of the following factors places Maggie Gardner at the greatest risk for developing anemia?
   a. Age at onset of pregnancy
   b. Presence of sickle cell trait
   c. Presence of autoimmune disorder
   d. Weight at the onset of pregnancy

3. _____ % to _____ % of women are affected by anemia during their pregnancy.

4. What complication do women with anemia experience at a higher rate than those without anemia?

5. The normal hematocrit level for pregnant women is:
   a. 25% to 29%.
   b. 28% to 35%.
   c. 35% to 40%.
   d. 37% to 47%.

6. What assessments specifically related to an anemia diagnosis need to be performed by the nurse at each visit?

7. When discussing dietary intake with Maggie Gardner, which of the following foods should be recommended as good sources of iron? Select all that apply.

   _____   Liver

   _____   Red meat

   _____   Citrus fruits

   _____   Leafy green vegetables

   _____   Butternut squash

   _____   Whole grain breads

8. When discussing iron supplementation with Maggie Gardner, which of the following instructions should be included? Select all that apply.

_____   Vitamin C (foods that contain vitamin C, such as orange juice, citrus fruits and strawberries) increases the absorption of iron.

_____   Milk can increase the absorption of iron.

_____   Stools may be black or dark green during iron therapy.

_____   Iron is best absorbed when taken during the early morning hours.

_____   Iron is best absorbed when taken on an empty stomach.

_____   Coffee and tea may decrease the absorption of iron supplements.

Exercise 2

Virtual Hospital Activity

20 minutes

Review Chapter 26 in the textbook.

1. A high risk pregnancy is one in which the life or health of _____ or _____ is

   jeopardized by a _____ coincidental with or unique to pregnancy.

- Sign in to work at Pacific View Regional Hospital for Period of Care 3. (*Note*: If you are already in the virtual hospital from a previous exercise, click on **Leave the Floor** and then on **Restart the Program** to get to the sign-in window.)
- From the Patient List, select Kelly Brady (Room 203), Maggie Gardner (Room 204), and Laura Wilson (Room 206).
- Click on **Go to Nurses' Station**.
- Click on **Chart**.
- For each of these three patients, open their chart and review the **History and Physical**.

2. For each of the patients below, list the things that place the patient at risk during her pregnancy.

Kelly Brady

Maggie Gardner

Laura Wilson

Review Box 26-1 in the textbook to answer the following questions.

3. The newborn of a patient who consumes a large amount of caffeine during pregnancy may experience

   _____.

4. The exact effects of alcohol in pregnancy are not known. However, it can result in _____,

   _____, _____, and _____.

5. According to the textbook, list three complications of a teenage pregnancy.

6. Primigravidas have a greater instance of what condition(s)? Select all that apply.

   _____ Ectopic pregnancy

   _____ Dystocia

   _____ Miscarriage

   _____ Preeclampsia

   _____ Abruptio placenta

7. The highest rate of premature and low-birth-weight babies is seen in:
   a. African Americans.
   b. Caucasians.
   c. Hispanics.
   d. Asian Americans.

Exercise 3

Virtual Hospital Activity

15 minutes

1. List three indications for the use of ultrasound.

2. What are two forms of ultrasound? When are they used?

- Sign in to work at Pacific View Regional Hospital for Period of Care 3. (*Note*: If you are already in the virtual hospital from a previous exercise, click on **Leave the Floor** and then on **Restart the Program** to get to the sign-in window.)
- From the Patient List, select Maggie Gardner (Room 204).
- Click on **Go to Nurses' Station**.
- Click on **Chart** and then on **204**.
- Click on **Diagnostic Reports**.

3. What type of ultrasound is Maggie Gardner having?

4. Based on the ultrasound findings, how large is her baby?

5. List three abnormalities found on Maggie Gardner's ultrasound in regard to the placenta.

6. What is the impression from Maggie Gardner's ultrasound in terms of the fetus and the placenta?

7. What are the recommendations regarding follow-up?

Exercise 4

Virtual Hospital Activity

20 minutes

1. What are the five items that are assessed on a biophysical profile?

2. Abnormalities in the amniotic fluid index are frequently associated with _____.

3. The biophysical profile is a reliable predictor of _____.

4. The normal score on a biophysical profile is _____.

- Sign in to work at Pacific View Regional Hospital for Period of Care 3. (*Note*: If you are already in the virtual hospital from a previous exercise, click on **Leave the Floor** and then on **Restart the Program** to get to the sign-in window.)
- From the Patient List, select Kelly Brady (Room 203).
- Click on **Go to Nurses' Station**.
- Click on **Chart** and then on **203**.
- Click on **Diagnostic Reports**.

5. What is the estimated gestational age of Kelly Brady's fetus?

6. What is the amniotic fluid index as indicated on the report?

7. How does this correlate with the normal index as listed in the textbook?

8. What is the score on the biophysical profile?

9. Based on the information that you have learned through your review of the textbook, what does this score indicate?

Nursing Care of the Pregnant Woman

Reading Assignment: Assessment and Health Promotion (Chapter 4)
Anatomy and Physiology of Pregnancy (Chapter 13)
Nursing Care of the Family During Pregnancy (Chapter 15)

Patients: Maggie Gardner, Room 204
Gabriela Valenzuela, Room 205
Laura Wilson, Room 206

Goal: To identify the variations found in the pregnant patient's assessment, including health risk behaviors and health promotion techniques to assist in the optimal outcome for the fetus.

Objectives:

- Discuss the variations in a pregnant patient's assessment findings.
- Identify health risks in pregnant patients.
- Explore health promotion interventions that can and should be completed by the nurse caring for those patients with high risk behaviors.

Exercise 1

Virtual Hospital Activity

45 minutes

After reviewing Chapter 4, Chapter 13, and Chapter 14, answer the following questions.

1. A nurse is reviewing the health history of a patient who is presently 14 weeks pregnant. The patient had an induced abortion at 8 weeks of gestation, delivered a stillborn child at 34 weeks, and has a living child who was born at 27 weeks of gestation. Using the gravidity, term, preterm, abortions, living children (GTPAL) obstetric history summary system, which of the following best describes this patient?
   a. 4-1-2-1-1
   b. 3-2-1-1-0
   c. 3-2-1-1-1
   d. 4-1-2-1-2

2. _____ is the hormone used in the detection of pregnancy.

3. When providing education to the pregnant woman, a nurse recognizes prenatal care should begin

   between _____ and _____ days after fertilization.

4. Identify the top four causes of death for women in the United States.

   _____ Diabetes mellitus

   _____ Heart disease

   _____ Cancer

   _____ Human immunodeficiency virus (HIV)

   _____ Complications of pregnancy

   _____ Stroke

   _____ Chronic lower respiratory disease

   _____ Kidney disease

5. Match each sign/symptom of pregnancy with the corresponding classification. Classifications may be used more than once.

Sign/Symptom of Pregnancy	Classification
_____ Amenorrhea	a. Presumptive
_____ Fetal heart tones	b. Probable
_____ Fetal movement	c. Positive
_____ Chadwick's sign	
_____ Human chorionic gonadotropin (hCG) in the urine	
_____ Ballottement	
_____ Quickening	
_____ Urinary frequency	

6. A nurse is providing education to a patient who is at 12 weeks of gestation. The patient asks how large her uterus is at this time. Which response best answers the patient's question?
   a. "Your uterus is the size of an apple."
   b. "Your uterus is the size of an egg."
   c. "Your uterus is the size of a grapefruit."
   d. "Your uterus is the size of a cantaloupe."

7. _____ Leukorrhea is a common finding in the pregnant woman with a bacterial infection. (True/False)

- Sign in to work at Pacific View Regional Hospital for Period of Care 1. (*Note*: If you are already in the virtual hospital from a previous exercise, click on **Leave the Floor** and then on **Restart the Program** to get to the sign-in window.)
- From the Patient List, select Maggie Gardner (Room 204).
- Click on **Go to Nurses' Station**.
- Click on **Chart** and then on **204**.
- Click on **Nursing Admission**.

8. Which of the following subjective presumptive indicators of pregnancy that apply to Maggie Gardner? Select all that apply.

    _____ Amenorrhea

    _____ Nausea/vomiting

    _____ Breast tenderness

    _____ Urinary frequency

    _____ Fatigue

    _____ Quickening

9. What is recorded as Maggie Gardner's last menstrual period (LMP)?

10. Using Nägele's Rule, calculate Maggie Gardner's estimated date of birth (EDB). Explain how you calculated this date.

11. Maggie Gardner is at _____ weeks of gestation.

- Click on **Return to Nurses' Station**.
- Click on **204** at the bottom of the screen.
- Click on **Take Vital Signs**.
- Click on **Patient Care** and then on **Physical Assessment**.
- Perform a focused abdominal assessment by clicking on the appropriate body system categories (yellow buttons) and body system subcategories (green buttons).

12. Maggie Gardner's heart rate is approximately 100 beats/min. Is this finding normal? What maternal heart rate changes are expected during pregnancy?

13. When reviewing the respiratory system of a pregnant woman, which of the following are normal findings? Select all that apply.

    _____ Slightly increased respiratory rate

    _____ Increased tidal volume

    _____ Unchanged total lung capacity

    _____ Increased inspiratory capacity

    _____ 30% increase in oxygen consumption

14. What probable and positive pregnancy indicators are found in Maggie Gardner's abdominal assessment?

Probable

Positive

15. What factors may be associated with variations in fundal height measurements?

- Still in Maggie Gardner's room, click on **Chart** at the top of the screen.
- Click on **204**.
- Click on the **Nursing Admission** tab and review.
- According to Chapter 4 of the textbook, there are many barriers to seeking health care. We see that this is true for Maggie Gardner. Continue reviewing the Nursing Admission section of her chart to answer the following questions regarding these barriers.

16. What are three barriers to seeking health care?

17. What barrier prevented Maggie Gardner from seeking health care?

Exercise 2

Virtual Hospital Activity

10 minutes

- Sign in to work at Pacific View Regional Hospital for Period of Care 3. (*Note*: If you are already in the virtual hospital from a previous exercise, click on **Leave the Floor** and then on **Restart the Program** to get to the sign-in window.)
- From the Patient List, select Laura Wilson (Room 206).
- Click on **Go to Nurses' Station**.
- Click on **Chart** and then on **206**.
- Review the **History and Physical** and the **Nursing Admission** to answer the following questions.

1. What was the clinician's perspective of Laura Wilson and her current life situation?

2. What was your impression of Laura Wilson?

- Click on **Return to Nurses' Station**.
- Click on **206** at the bottom of the screen.
- Click on **Patient Care** and then on **Nurse-Client Interactions**.
- Select and view the video titled **1530: Discharge Planning**. (*Note:* Check the virtual clock to see whether enough time has elapsed. You can use the fast-forward feature to advance the time by 2-minute intervals if the video is not yet available. Then click again on **Patient Care** and **Nurse-Client Interactions** to refresh the screen.)

3. What does Laura Wilson say that indicates that she may not understand HIV or is in denial that it is truly a medical concern?

- Click on **Chart** and then on **206**.
- Click on **Consultations** and review the Psychiatric Consult.

4. From your review of the 1530 video and the Psychiatric Consult notes, what areas of health education (health promotion) need to be the focus for Laura Wilson?

Exercise 3

Virtual Hospital Activity

20 minutes

The head-to-toe assessment is a key part of obtaining data, both subjective and objective, from our patients. The following exercise will walk you through a head-to-toe assessment on a pregnant patient. The goal of this exercise is to identify findings that are abnormal and recognize those that are pregnancy-related.

- Sign in to work at Pacific View Regional Hospital for Period of Care 2. (*Note:* If you are already in the virtual hospital from a previous exercise, click on **Leave the Floor** and then on **Restart the Program** to get to the sign-in window.)
- From the Patient List, select Gabriela Valenzuela (Room 205).
- Click on **Go to Nurses' Station** and then on **205** at the bottom of the screen.
- Click on **Patient Care** and then on **Physical Assessment**.
- Complete a focused assessment by clicking on the various body system categories (yellow buttons) and body system subcategories (green buttons).

1. Record any abnormal findings or any pregnancy-related findings below.

    a. Head & Neck

    b. Chest

    c. Back & Spine

    d. Upper Extremities

    e. Abdomen

    f. Pelvic

    g. Lower Extremities

2. What is the nurse's responsibility to the patient on return visits?

3. Identify five areas in which women should be educated in order to maintain a healthy life.

4. According to Box 4-11 in your textbook, pelvic examinations are recommended

    _____ for women ages _____ to _____ years old. They are to be started

    _____ or when a female _____, whichever comes first.

LESSON 7 ―――――――――――――――――――――

Nursing Care During Labor and Birth

―――――――――――――――――――――――――――――――

Reading Assignment: Nursing Care of the Family During Labor (Chapter 19)

Patients: Dorothy Grant, Room 201
Gabriela Valenzuela, Room 205
Laura Wilson, Room 206

Goal: To demonstrate an understanding of the normal labor and birth process.

Objectives:

- Assess and identify signs and symptoms present in each phase of the first stage of labor.
- Describe appropriate nursing care for the patient in the first stage of labor.

Exercise 1

Virtual Hospital Activity

20 minutes

- Sign in to work at Pacific View Regional Hospital for Period of Care 1. (*Note*: If you are already in the virtual hospital from a previous exercise, click on **Leave the Floor** and then on **Restart the Program** to get to the sign-in window.)
- From the Patient List, select Dorothy Grant (Room 201).
- Click on **Go to Nurses' Station**.
- Click on **Chart** and then on **201**.
- Click on **Nurse's Notes** and review the entry for Wednesday 0730.

1. List the findings from Dorothy Grant's most recent cervical examination.

- Click on **Return to Nurses' Station**.
- Click on **EPR**.
- Click on **Login**.
- Select **201** from the Patient drop-down menu and **Obstetrics** from the Category drop-down menu.

2. What was the recorded frequency and duration of Dorothy Grant's contractions at 0700?

- Now select **Vital Signs** from the Category drop-down menu.

3. What was Dorothy Grant's recorded pain level at 0700?

Consult Table 19-1 in your textbook.

4. At this time, in which phase of the first stage of labor is Dorothy Grant?

5. For each specific assessment listed below, compare the typical findings for latent labor with Dorothy Grant's current condition.

Assessment	Typical Findings for Latent Labor	Findings for Dorothy Grant
Cervical dilation		
Contraction frequency		
Contraction duration		
Contraction strength		

6. List the typical behaviors of the latent phase of labor.

- Click on **Exit EPR**.
- Click on **201** at the bottom of the screen.
- Click on **Patient Care** and then on **Nurse-Client Interactions**.
- Select and view the video titled **0810: Monitoring/Patient Support**. (*Note:* Check the virtual clock to see whether enough time has elapsed. You can use the fast-forward feature to advance the time by 2-minute intervals if the video is not yet available. Then click again on **Patient Care** and **Nurse-Client Interactions** to refresh the screen.)

7. Based on the video interaction, which of the following accurately describe Dorothy Grant? Select all that apply.

_____ Excited

_____ Thoughts center on self, labor, and baby

_____ Some apprehension

_____ Pain controlled fairly well

_____ Alert

_____ Follows directions readily

_____ Open to instructions

Exercise 2

Virtual Hospital Activity

20 minutes

Read the sections on Nursing Interventions During Labor and Supportive Care During Labor and Birth in your textbook.

- Sign in to work at Pacific View Regional Hospital for Period of Care 2. (*Note*: If you are already in the virtual hospital from a previous exercise, click on **Leave the Floor** and then on **Restart the Program** to get to the sign-in window.)
- From the Patient List, select Gabriela Valenzuela (Room 205).
- Click on **Go to Nurses' Station**.
- Click on **Chart** and then on **205**.
- Click on **Nurse's Notes** and scroll to review the note for Wednesday at 0800.

1. What was Gabriela Valenzuela's condition at this time? What phase of labor was she experiencing?

2. As Gabriela Valenzuela progresses in labor, which phase will she enter next?

3. According to Box 19-10 in the textbook, list five common interventions applied during the second stage of labor.

- Click on **Return to Nurses' Station**.
- Use the fast-forward feature to advance the clock to 1140.
- Click on **Chart** and then on **205**.
- Click on **Nurse's Notes** and review the entry for Wednesday 1140.

4. How is Gabriela Valenzuela tolerating labor at this time? Do you believe she has entered the active phase of labor?

5. How could you determine for certain which phase of labor Gabriela Valenzuela is currently experiencing?

- Click on **Return to Nurses' Station**.
- Click on **205** at the bottom of the screen.
- Click on **Patient Care** and then on **Nurse-Client Interactions**.
- Select and view the video titled: **1140: Intervention—Bleeding, Comfort**. (*Note:* Check the virtual clock to see whether enough time has elapsed. You can use the fast-forward feature to advance the time by 2-minute intervals if the video is not yet available. Then click again on **Patient Care** and **Nurse-Client Interactions** to refresh the screen.)

6. During the video interaction, which of the following interventions were suggested or implemented by the nurse? Select all that apply.

_____ Limit assessment techniques to between contractions

_____ Assist patient to cope with contractions

_____ Encourage patient to help her maintain breathing techniques

_____ Use comfort measures

_____ Assist with position changes

_____ Offer encouragement and praise

_____ Keep patient aware of progress

_____ Offer analgesics as ordered

_____ Check bladder; encourage voiding

_____ Give oral care; offer fluids, food, ice chips as ordered

- Click on **Patient Care** and then on **Nurse-Client Interactions**.
- Select and view the video titled **1155: Evaluation—Comfort Measures**. (*Note:* Check the virtual clock to see whether enough time has elapsed. You can use the fast-forward feature to advance the time by 2-minute intervals if the video is not available. Then click again on **Patient Care** and **Nurse-Client Interactions** to refresh the screen.)

7. During the video interaction, which of the following interventions were suggested or implemented by the nurse and/or Gabriela Valenzuela's husband? Select all that apply.

_____ Limit assessment techniques to between contractions

_____ Assist patient to cope with contractions

_____ Encourage patient to help her maintain breathing techniques

_____ Use comfort measures

_____ Assist with position changes

_____ Offer encouragement and praise

_____ Keep patient aware of progress

_____ Offer analgesics as ordered

_____ Check bladder; encourage voiding

_____ Give oral care; offer fluids, food, ice chips as ordered

Exercise 3

Virtual Hospital Activity

45 minutes

Let's jump ahead to Period of Care 4. Remember, you are not able to visit patients during this shift, but you have access to all patient records. First, we'll review Dorothy Grant's status.

- Sign in to work at Pacific View Regional Hospital for Period of Care 4. (*Note:* If you are already in the virtual hospital from a previous exercise, click on **Leave the Floor** and then on **Restart the Program** to get to the sign-in window.)
- From the Nurses' Station, click on **EPR** and then on **Login**.
- Select **201** from the Patient drop-down menu and **Obstetrics** from the Category drop-down menu.
- Use the arrows at the bottom of the screen to review the entries for Wednesday 1800 and 1815.

1. What are the findings from Dorothy Grant's cervical examination at 1815?

2. At this time, which phase of the first stage of labor is Dorothy Grant experiencing?

3. Using Table 19-1 in your textbook, complete the table below, listing typical findings for each assessment in the transition phase of the first stage of labor.

Assessment	Typical Findings
Cervical dilation	
Contraction frequency	
Contraction duration	
Contraction strength	

4. List the typical behaviors seen in patients experiencing the transition phase of labor.

- Click on **Exit EPR**.
- Click on **Chart** and then on **201** for Dorothy Grant's chart.
- Click on **Nurse's Notes**.
- Read the notes recorded at 1800, 1815, and 1830 on Wednesday.

5. Based on information recorded in the EPR and Nurse's Notes, which of the following behaviors did Dorothy Grant exhibit during the transition phase of labor? Select all that apply.

_____   Severe pain

_____   Frustration; fear of loss of control

_____   Writhing with contractions

_____   Nausea/vomiting

_____   Perspiration

_____   Shaking or tremors

_____   Feeling the need to defecate

_____   Hyperesthesia

Now let's review Laura Wilson's status.

- Click on **Return to Nurses' Station**.
- Click on **EPR** and then on **Login**.
- Select **206** from the Patient drop-down menu and **Vital Signs** from the Category drop-down menu.

6. Below, record Laura Wilson's assessment findings from 1815 on Wednesday.

Pain location

Pain intensity

- Now select **Obstetrics** from the Category drop-down menu.

7. Below, record Laura Wilson's 1830 assessment findings.

Contraction frequency

Contraction duration

- Use the arrows at the bottom of the screen to view other Obstetrics entries until you locate the results of Laura Wilson's most recent cervical examination.

8. When was Laura Wilson's most recent cervical examination performed? What were the results?

- Click on **Exit EPR**.
- Click on **Chart** and then on **206**.
- Click **Nurse's Notes**.
- Scroll to the note for Wednesday at 1830.

9. According to this note, what event occurred at 1815?

Read the information on Assessment of Amniotic Membranes and Fluid in your textbook. Also read the information in Box 19-1.

10. List the immediate nursing actions appropriate for the situation you identified in question 9.

11. According to the Nurse's Notes and your textbook recommendations, did Laura Wilson's nurse handle this situation appropriately? Explain.

12. Based only on the information you have learned about Laura Wilson during this activity, write the nursing diagnosis that you consider to be of highest priority for her at this time.

13. List several nursing interventions for the nursing diagnosis you wrote in question 12.

Management of Discomfort

Reading Assignment: Pain Management (Chapter 17)

Patients: Kelly Brady, Room 203
Gabriela Valenzuela, Room 205
Laura Wilson, Room 206

Goal: To demonstrate an understanding of the management of discomfort during the normal labor and birth process.

Objectives:

- Assess and identify factors that influence pain perception.
- Describe selected nonpharmacologic and pharmacologic measures for pain management during labor and birth.

Exercise 1

Virtual Hospital Activity

20 minutes

- Sign in to work at Pacific View Regional Hospital for Period of Care 1. (*Note*: If you are already in the virtual hospital from a previous exercise, click on **Leave the Floor** and then on **Restart the Program** to get to the sign-in window.)
- From the Patient List, select Laura Wilson (Room 206).
- Click on **Get Report**.

1. What is Laura Wilson's condition when you assume care for her, according to the change-of-shift report?

- Click on **Go to Nurses' Station**.
- Click on **206** at the bottom of the screen.
- Read the Initial Observations.

2. What is your impression of Laura Wilson's condition?

- Click on **Patient Care** and then on **Nurse-Client Interactions**.
- Select and view the video titled **0730: Patient Assessment**. (*Note:* Check the virtual clock to see whether enough time has elapsed. You can use the fast-forward feature to advance the time by 2-minute intervals if the video is not yet available. Then click again on **Patient Care** and **Nurse-Client Interactions** to refresh the screen.)

3. What is Laura Wilson's assessment of her current condition? How does this compare with the information you received from the shift report and the Initial Observations summary?

- Click on **Chart** and then on **206**.
- Click on **Nursing Admission**.

4. List Laura Wilson's admission diagnoses.

5. What is your perception of Laura Wilson's behavior? What data did you collect during this exercise that led you to this perception?

6. Think about the following questions and then discuss your ideas with your classmates. Do your personal values and beliefs contribute to your perception of Laura Wilson's behavior? If so, how? What nursing interventions might help to overcome your personal biases when dealing with Laura Wilson?

Read the section on Factors Influencing Pain Response in your textbook.

• Continue reviewing Laura Wilson's **Nursing Admission** form as needed to answer question 7.

7. Each woman's pain during childbirth is unique and is influenced by a variety of factors. For each factor listed below, explain how that factor influences pain perception (in the middle column). Then, in the right column, list data from Laura Wilson's Nursing Admission that support how that factor might relate to her particular pain perception.

Factor	Typical Effect on Pain Perception	Laura Wilson's Supporting Data
Anxiety		
Previous experience		
Childbirth preparation		
Support		

Exercise 2

Virtual Hospital Activity

45 minutes

- Sign in to work at Pacific View Regional Hospital for Period of Care 2. (*Note*: If you are already in the virtual hospital from a previous exercise, click on **Leave the Floor** and then on **Restart the Program** to get to the sign-in window.)
- From the Patient List, select Gabriela Valenzuela (Room 205).

Read the section on Nonpharmacologic Pain Management in your textbook.

1. According to Box 17-2, identify nonpharmacologic sensory stimulation strategies that can be used to provide pain relief to the laboring woman.

2. During labor a woman may drink tea to promote relaxation and help with hydration. What type of tea may be recommended?
   a. Lemon balm
   b. Peppermint
   c. Chamomile
   d. Ginger

3. A nurse is caring for a laboring patient. Which of the following breathing techniques is recommended during the transition phase of labor?
   a. Pattern-paced breathing
   b. Deep-cleanse breathing
   c. Slow-paced breathing
   d. Rapid-paced breathing

4. Touch can communicate _____, _____, and _____. When using

   touch, it is important to determine the _____. Head, hand, back, and

   foot massage may be very effective in _____ and

   _____.

- Click on **Get Report**.

5. Is Gabriela Valenzuela in labor at this time? Give a rationale for your answer.

- Click **Go to Nurses' Station**.
- Click on **205** at the bottom of the screen.
- Click on **Patient Care** and then on **Nurse-Client Interactions**.
- Select and view the video titled **1140: Intervention—Bleeding, Comfort**. (*Note:* Check the virtual clock to see whether enough time has elapsed. You can use the fast-forward feature to advance the time by 2-minute intervals if the video is not yet available. Then click again on **Patient Care** and **Nurse-Client Interactions** to refresh the screen.)
- Click on **Chart** and then on **205**.
- Click on **Nurse's Notes** and review the note for Wednesday at 1140.

6. How is Gabriela Valenzuela tolerating labor at this time?

7. What pain interventions does the nurse implement at this time?

8. What is the action of the drug administered by the nurse?

Let's begin the process for preparing Gabriela Valenzuela's fentanyl dose.

- Click on **Return to Room 205**.
- Click on **Medication Room**.
- Next, click on **MAR** and then on tab **205**.
- Scroll down to the PRN Medication Administration Record for Wednesday.

9. What is the ordered dose of fentanyl?

- Click on **Return to Medication Room**.
- Click on **Automated System**.
- Click on **Log In**.
- In box 1, select **Gabriela Valenzuela, 205**.
- In box 2, select **Automated System Drawer A-F**.
- Click on **Open Drawer**.

- Click on **Fentanyl citrate** and then on **Put Medication on Tray**.
- Click on **Close Drawer** and then on **View Medication Room**.
- Click on **Preparation**.
- Click on **Prepare** next to fentanyl citrate and follow the Preparation Wizard prompts to complete the preparation of Gabriela Valenzuela's fentanyl dose. When the Wizard stops requesting information, click on **Finish**.
- Click on **Return to Medication Room**.
- Click on **205** at the bottom of the screen to go to the patient's room.

10. What additional assessments must be completed before you give Gabriela Valenzuela's medication?

11. Why is it important to check Gabriela Valenzuela's respirations before giving the dose of fentanyl?

12. What safety precautions should be in effect for Gabriela Valenzuela after she receives this dose of fentanyl?

- Click on **Patient Care** and then on **Medication Administration**.
- Click on **Review Your Medications** and verify the accuracy of your preparation.
- Click on **Return to Room 205**.
- Next, click the down arrow next to **Select** and choose **Administer**.
- Follow the Administration Wizard prompts to administer Gabriela Valenzuela's fentanyl dose. Click **Yes** when asked whether to document this administration in the MAR.
- When the Wizard stops asking questions, click on **Finish**.
- Click on **Patient Care** and then on **Nurse-Client Interactions**.
- Select and view the video titled: **1155: Evaluation—Comfort Measures**. (*Note:* Check the virtual clock to see whether enough time has elapsed. You can use the fast-forward feature to advance the time by 2-minute intervals if the video is not yet available. Then click again on **Patient Care** and **Nurse-Client Interactions** to refresh the screen.)

13. How effective were the interventions you identified in question 7?

14. Gabriela Valenzuela is experiencing _____. _____ is

    responsible for the dizziness as well as other side effects, including

    _____, _____, and

    _____.

15. What interventions does the nurse suggest to deal with this problem? List other interventions described
    in your textbook.

At the end of the 1155 video, Gabriela Valenzuela states that she "doesn't want any needles" in her back.
Read the section on Epidural or Spinal Anesthesia in your textbook.

16. What could you tell Gabriela Valenzuela to help her make an informed decision about anesthesia for
    labor? Below, list advantages and disadvantages of epidural anesthesia.

Advantages   **Disadvantages**

Before leaving this period of care, let's see how you did preparing and administering the patient's
medication.

- Click on **Leave the Floor**.
- Click on **Look at Your Preceptor's Evaluation**.
- Click on **Medication Scorecard** and review the evaluation. How did you do?

Exercise 3

Virtual Hospital Activity

15 minutes

Read the section on General Anesthesia in your textbook.

• Sign in to work at Pacific View Regional Hospital for Period of Care 4. (*Note*: If you are already in the virtual hospital from a previous exercise, click on **Leave the Floor** and then on **Restart the Program** to get to the sign-in window.)
• From the Nurses' Station, click on **Chart** and then on **203** for Kelly Brady's chart. (*Remember:* You are not able to visit patients or administer medications during Period of Care 4. You are able to review patient records only.)
• Click on **Nurse's Notes**.
• Scroll to the entry for 1730 on Wednesday.

1. Why does the anesthesiologist plan to use general anesthesia during Kelly Brady's cesarean birth? (*Hint*: Read the section on Contraindications to Subarachnoid and Epidural Blocks in your textbook.)

2. Why is Kelly Brady upset about receiving general anesthesia for her surgery?

• Click on **Physician's Orders** and review the entry for Wednesday at 1540.

3. What preoperative medications are ordered for Kelly Brady?

• Click on **Return to Nurses' Station**.
• Click on the **Drug** icon in the lower left corner of your screen to access the Drug Guide.
• Use the search box or the scroll bar to read about each of the drugs you listed in question 3.

4. All of the ordered preoperative medications are given to help prevent aspiration pneumonia. Using information from the Drug Guide and from the section on General Anesthesia in your textbook, match each of the medications below with the description of how it specifically works to prevent aspiration pneumonia.

Medication	Mechanism of Action
_____ Sodium citrate/citric acid (Bicitra)	a. Decreases the production of gastric acid
_____ Metoclopramide (Reglan)	b. Prevents nausea and vomiting and accelerates gastric emptying
_____ Ranitidine (Zantac)	c. Neutralizes acidic stomach contents

5. During general anesthesia, a short-acting barbiturate or ketamine is administered to

_____. A muscle relaxer is then given to _____

_____. A low concentration of a volatile halogenated agent may be

administered to _____.

6. How would you expect general anesthesia to affect Kelly Brady's baby? Why?

LESSON

9

Hypertensive Disorders in Pregnancy

Reading Assignment: Hypertensive Disorders (Chapter 27)

Patient: Kelly Brady, Room 203

Goal: To demonstrate an understanding of the identification and management of selected hypertensive complications of pregnancy.

Objectives:

- Assess and identify signs and symptoms present in the patient with severe preeclampsia.
- Explain how common signs and symptoms present in the patient with severe preeclampsia relate to the underlying pathophysiology of the disease.
- Identify the patient who has developed HELLP syndrome.
- Describe routine nursing care for the patient with severe preeclampsia who is receiving magnesium sulfate.

Exercise 1

Virtual Hospital Activity

15 minutes

- Sign in to work at Pacific View Regional Hospital for Period of Care 3. (*Note:* If you are already in the virtual hospital from a previous exercise, click on **Leave the Floor** and then on **Restart the Program** to get to the sign-in window.)
- From the Patient List, select Kelly Brady (Room 203).
- Click on **Go to Nurses' Station**.
- Click on **Chart** and then on **203**.
- Click on **History and Physical**.

1. What was Kelly Brady's admission diagnosis?

2. Use Kelly Brady's History and Physical and Chapter 27 in your textbook to complete the table below.

Sign/Symptom	Preeclampsia	Severe Preeclampsia	Kelly Brady on Admission
Blood pressure			
Proteinuria			
Headache			
Visual problems			
Epigastric pain			

- Click on **Physician's Orders** and scroll to the admitting physician's orders on Tuesday at 1030.

3. What tests/procedures did Kelly Brady's physician order to confirm the diagnosis of severe preeclampsia?

- Click on **Physician's Notes** and scroll to the note for Wednesday at 0730.

4. What subjective and objective data are recorded here that would support the diagnosis of severe preeclampsia?

Kelly Brady's 24-hour urine collection was completed and sent to the lab at 1230.

- Click on **Laboratory Reports**.
- Scroll to find the Wednesday 1230 results.

5. Below, record the results of Kelly Brady's 24-hour urine collection.

6. Now list all the data you have collected during this exercise that confirm Kelly Brady's diagnosis of severe preeclampsia.

7. Worldwide, _____ of maternal deaths can be attributed to preeclampsia and eclampsia.
   a. 5% to 10%
   b. 10% to 15%
   c. 15% to 18%
   d. 18% to 20%

Exercise 2

Virtual Hospital Activity

10 minutes

- Sign in to work at Pacific View Regional Hospital for Period of Care 1. (*Note*: If you are already in the virtual hospital from a previous exercise, click on **Leave the Floor** and then on **Restart the Program** to get to the sign-in window.)
- From the Patient List, select Kelly Brady (Room 203).
- Click on **Go to Nurses' Station**.
- Click on **203** at the bottom of the screen.
- Click on **Take Vital Signs**.

1. Record Kelly Brady's vital signs for 0730 below.

- Click on **Patient Care** and then on **Physical Assessment**.
- Complete an assessment by clicking on the various body system categories (yellow buttons) and body system subcategories (green buttons) as specified in question 2.

2. Record your findings from the focused assessment of Kelly Brady in the table below.

Body System Categories	Body System Subcategories	Kelly Brady's Findings
Head & Neck	Sensory	
Head & Neck	Neurologic	
Chest	Respiratory	
Abdomen	Gastrointestinal	
Lower Extremities	Neurologic	

3. The main pathogenic factor in the woman with preeclampsia is not _____,

   but _____, as a result of _____ and _____.

4. Match each of the signs/symptoms below with the preeclampsia-associated pathology. Some pathologies will be used more than once.

Signs/Symptoms	Preeclampsia-Associated Pathology
_____ Blurred vision/scotomata	a. Generalized vasoconstriction
_____ Headache	b. Glomerular damage
_____ Epigastric or right upper quadrant abdominal pain	c. Retinal arteriolar spasms
	d. Hepatic microemboli; liver damage
_____ 4+ reflexes/clonus	e. Cortical brain spasms
_____ Elevated blood pressure	
_____ Proteinuria/oliguria	

Exercise 3

Virtual Hospital Activity

20 minutes

- Sign in to work at Pacific View Regional Hospital for Period of Care 3. (*Note*: If you are already in the virtual hospital from a previous exercise, click on **Leave the Floor** and then on **Restart the Program** to get to the sign-in window.)
- From the Patient List, select Kelly Brady (Room 203).
- Click on **Go to Nurses' Station**.

Read about HELLP syndrome in your textbook.

1. Why do you think Kelly Brady had blood drawn at 1230 for an aspartate aminotransferase (AST) measurement and a platelet count?

- Click on **Chart** and then on **203**.
- Click on **Laboratory Reports**.
- Scroll to the report for Wednesday 1230 to locate the results of these tests.

2. Complete the table below based on your review of the Laboratory Reports and Table 27-3 in your textbook.

Test	Wed 1230 Result	Normal (Nonpregnant) Value	Value in HELLP
Platelet count			
AST			

- Click on **Return to Nurses' Station**.
- Click on **Patient List**.
- Click on **Get Report** for Kelly Brady.

3. Why has Kelly Brady been transferred to Labor and Delivery?

4. The nurses caring for Kelly Brady must have an understanding of HELLP syndrome. Which of the following statements concerning the illness are correct? Select all that apply.

_____   Women with HELLP syndrome will demonstrate significant increases in blood pressure.

_____   HELLP syndrome is most common in the third trimester and postpartum period.

_____   Hemoglobin levels in the patient experiencing HELLP syndrome will be elevated.

_____   Hematocrit levels in the patient experiencing HELLP syndrome will be decreased.

_____   Low platelet count values are consistent with HELLP syndrome.

_____   HELLP syndrome is a variant of severe preeclampsia.

5. What type of woman is most likely to develop HELLP syndrome? Which of these characteristics is true of Kelly Brady?

- Click on **Return to Nurses' Station.**
- Use the fast-forward feature to advance the virtual clock to 1530.
- Click on **Chart** and then on **203**.
- Click on **Physician's Notes** and review the note for Wednesday at 1530.

6. What is the physician's plan of care for Kelly Brady, in light of the HELLP syndrome diagnosis?

Assume that you will be the nurse caring for Kelly Brady after her surgery while she is receiving magnesium sulfate. Read about this medication in your textbook and then answer question 7.

7. All of the assessments/interventions listed below are part of routine nursing care for a patient with severe preeclampsia. Which of these activities are performed specifically to assess for magnesium toxicity? Select all that apply.

_____ Measuring/recording urine output

_____ Measuring proteinuria using urine dipstick

_____ Monitoring liver enzyme levels and platelet count

_____ Monitoring for headache, visual disturbances, and epigastric pain

_____ Assessing for decreased level of consciousness

_____ Assessing deep tendon reflexes (DTRs)

_____ Weighing daily to assess for edema

_____ Monitoring vital signs, especially respiratory rate

_____ Dimming room lights and maintaining a quiet environment

8. A nurse administering magnesium sulfate to Kelly Brady must have which of the following antidotes on hand?
a. Narcan
b. Calcium gluconate
c. Atropine sulfate
d. Naloxone

9. _____ Women with HELLP syndrome frequently do not manifest symptoms consistent with severe preeclampsia. (True/False)

10. When caring for Kelly Brady, a nurse recognizes that perinatal mortality associated with HELLP syndrome is:
a. less than 5%.
b. 7% to 34%.
c. 20% to 34%.
d. 30% to 40%.

LESSON 10

Antepartum Hemorrhagic Disorders

Reading Assignment: Hemorrhagic Disorders in Pregnancy (Chapter 28)

Patient: Gabriela Valenzuela, Room 205

Goal: To demonstrate an understanding of the identification and management of selected hemorrhagic complications of pregnancy.

Objectives:

- Identify appropriate interventions for managing abruptio placentae.
- Differentiate between the symptoms related to an abruptio placentae and those related to a placenta previa.
- Plan and evaluate essential patient education during the acute phase of diagnosis.

Exercise 1

Virtual Hospital Activity

30 minutes

- Sign in to work at Pacific View Regional Hospital for Period of Care 1. (*Note*: If you are already in the virtual hospital from a previous exercise, click on **Leave the Floor** and then on **Restart the Program** to get to the sign-in window.)
- From the Patient List, select Gabriela Valenzuela (Room 205).
- Click on **Go to Nurses' Station**.
- Click on **Chart** and then on **205**.
- Click on **Emergency Department**.

1. What brought Gabriela Valenzuela to the Emergency Department (ED)? How long had she waited to actually come to the ED? What was the deciding factor in her coming to the ED?

Read about the incidence and etiology of Late Pregnancy Bleeding in your textbook.

2. Other than a motor vehicle accident (MVA), what could result in or increase the risk for having an abruptio placentae?

3. Differential diagnosis is very important when you are confronted with clinical manifestations that could be evidence of more than one process. Compare and contrast abruptio placentae with placenta previa.

Characteristic/Complication	Abruptio Placentae	Placenta Previa
Bleeding		
Shock		
Coagulopathy (DIC)		
Uterine tonicity		
Tenderness/pain		
Placenta findings		
Fetal heart rate effects		

4. Based on your review of the ED record, what grade of abruption does Gabriela Valenzuela have?
   a. Grade 1
   b. Grade 2
   c. Grade 3

- Click on **Return to Nurses' Station**.
- Click on **205** at the bottom of the screen.
- Click on **Patient Care** and then on **Nurse-Client Interactions**.
- Select and view the video titled **0740: Patient Teaching—Fetal Monitoring**. (*Note:* Check the virtual clock to see whether enough time has elapsed. You can use the fast-forward feature to advance the time by 2-minute intervals if the video is not yet available. Then click again on **Patient Care** and **Nurse-Client Interactions** to refresh the screen.)

5. Once Gabriela Valenzuela is admitted to the floor, what are her and her husband's concerns? What does the nurse include in her teaching to alleviate those concerns?

Gabriela Valenzuela is at increased risk for early delivery as a result of the abdominal trauma she suffered and the subsequent occurrence of abruptio placentae. She is currently manifesting signs and symptoms of early labor. According to the Physician's Orders, she was given a dose of betamethasone and this was to be repeated in 12 hours.

6. What is the purpose of the administration of betamethasone in this patient's scenario?

- Click on **MAR** and then on **205**. Review the betamethasone dosage to be given to Gabriela Valenzuela.
- Click on **Return to Room 205** and then on **Medication Room**.
- Click on **Unit Dosage** and then on drawer **205**.
- Click on **Betamethasone** and then on **Put Medication on Tray**.
- Click on **Close Drawer** and then on **View Medication Room**.
- Click on **Preparation**.
- Click on **Prepare** next to Betamethasone and follow the Preparation Wizard's prompts to complete the preparation of Gabriela Valenzuela's betamethasone.
- When the Wizard stops asking questions, click on **Finish**.
- Click on **Return to Medication Room**.
- Click on **205** at the bottom of the screen to return to the patient's room.
- Click on **Patient Care** and then on **Medication Administration**.
- Click on **Review Your Medications**.
- Click on the tab marked **Prepared**.

7. According to the textbox on the right side of your screen, what is the medication name and dosage that you have prepared for Gabriela Valenzuela?

8. How many milligrams are you giving to Gabriela Valenzuela based on the answer to the previous question? Is this the correct dosage based on the MAR?

- Click on **Return to Room 205**.
- Click on the **Drug** icon in the left-hand corner of the screen.
- To read about betamethasone, either type the drug name in the search box or scroll through the alphabetic list of medications at the top of the screen.

9. Based on the information provided in the Drug Guide, what is the indication and dosage for this medication in regard to pregnant adults?

10. When preparing to administer betamethasone, which of the following areas need to be assessed in Gabriela Valenzuela's history? Select all that apply.

_____   Assess for kidney disease

_____   Assess for allergies/hypersensitivity to corticosteroids and sulfate

_____   Assess for a history of diabetes

_____   Determine whether the patient is on digoxin

_____   Assess baseline heart rate

_____   Assess baseline blood pressure

11. Now review the information regarding the administration of this medication. What are three things that need to be taken into consideration when giving this medication in the injection form?

12. What are the Six Rights of medication administration as they relate to the patient?

You are now ready to complete the medication administration.

- Click on **Return to Room 205**.
- Click on **Check Armband**.
- Select **Administer** from the drop-down menu to the left of Betamethasone.
- Follow the Medication Wizard's prompts to administer Gabriela Valenzuela's betamethasone. Click **Yes** when asked whether to document the injection in the MAR.
- When the Wizard is finished asking questions, click on **Finish**.
- Now click on **Patient Care** and then on **Nurse-Client Interactions**.
- Select and view the video titled **0805: Patient Teaching—Abruption**. (*Note:* Check the virtual clock to see whether enough time has elapsed. You can use the fast-forward feature to advance the time by 2-minute intervals if the video is not yet available. Then click again on **Patient Care** and **Nurse-Client Interactions** to refresh the screen.)

13. According to the video, what will help increase the oxygen supply to the baby and prevent further separation of the placenta?

* Click on **Leave the Floor**.
* Click on **Look at Your Preceptor's Evaluation**.
* Click on **Medication Scorecard** and review the evaluation. How did you do?

Exercise 2

Virtual Hospital Activity

15 minutes

* Sign in to work at Pacific View Regional Hospital for Period of Care 2. (*Note*: If you are already in the virtual hospital from a previous exercise, click on **Leave the Floor** and then on **Restart the Program** to get to the sign-in window.)
* From the Patient List, select Gabriela Valenzuela (Room 205).
* Click on **Go to Nurses' Station**.
* Click on **Chart** and then on **205**.
* Click on **Diagnostic Reports**.

Gabriela Valenzuela had an ultrasound done on Tuesday to determine the source of the bleeding.

1. What were the findings on the ultrasound?

* Click on the **Laboratory Reports**.

2. What were Gabriela Valenzuela's hemoglobin and hematocrit levels on Tuesday? How do these findings compare with Wednesday's report? Has there been a significant change?

3. What clinical manifestations would indicate a worsening in the condition of either the patient or the fetus? (*Hint:* Review your textbook regarding outcomes, diagnosis, and management.)

- Click on **Return to Nurses' Station**.
- Click on **EPR** and then on **Login**.
- Select **205** from the Patient drop-down menu and **Vital Signs** from the Category drop-down menu.
- Use the arrows at the bottom of the screen to review the vital sign findings over the last 12 hours.

4. From 0000 Wednesday until 1200 Wednesday, would you consider Gabriela Valenzuela's condition stable or unstable? State the rationale for your answer.

- Click on **Exit EPR**.
- Click on **205** at the bottom of the screen.
- Click on **Patient Care** and then on **Nurse-Client Interactions**.
- Select and view the video titled **1140: Intervention—Bleeding, Comfort**. Take notes as you watch and listen. (*Note:* Check the virtual clock to see whether enough time has elapsed. You can use the fast-forward feature to advance the time by 2-minute intervals if the video is not yet available. Then click again on **Patient Care** and **Nurse-Client Interactions** to refresh the screen.)
- Click on **Chart** and then on **205**.
- Click on **Nurse's Notes** and review the note for Wednesday at 1140.

5. What happened that elicited the interaction between the patient and the nurse?

6. What actions did the nurse take during the interaction?

Exercise 3

Virtual Hospital Activity

20 minutes

- Sign in to work at Pacific View Regional Hospital for Period of Care 3. (*Note*: If you are already in the virtual hospital from a previous exercise, click on **Leave the Floor** and then on **Restart the Program** to get to the sign-in window.)
- From the Patient List, select Gabriela Valenzuela (Room 205).
- Click on **Go to Nurses' Station**.
- Click on **Kardex** and then on tab **205**.

1. What problem areas have been identified by the nurse related to Gabriela Valenzuela's diagnosis?

2. What is the focus of the outcomes related to the above mentioned problems?

3. Using correct North American Nursing Diagnosis Association (NANDA) nursing diagnosis terminology, list four possible nursing diagnoses appropriate for Gabriela Valenzuela at this time.

- Click on **Return to Nurses' Station**.
- Click on **Chart** and then on **205**.
- Click on **Patient Education**.

4. According to the Patient Education sheet in Gabriela Valenzuela's chart, what are the educational goals related to the patient's diagnosis?

- Click on **Nurse's Notes**.

5. What education has been completed by the nurses through Period of Care 3? Include the time and topics discussed.

6. What are some barriers to learning that the nurse may confront with this patient?

7. How can the nurse overcome each of these barriers?

Endocrine and Metabolic Disorders

Reading Assignment: Endocrine and Metabolic Disorders (Chapter 29)

Patient: Stacey Crider, Room 202

Goal: To demonstrate an understanding of the identification and management of selected endocrine complications of pregnancy.

Objectives:

- Identify appropriate interventions for controlling hyperglycemia in a patient with gestational diabetes mellitus (GDM).
- Correctly administer insulin to a patient with GDM.
- Plan and evaluate essential patient teaching for a patient with GDM.

Exercise 1

Virtual Hospital Activity

20 minutes

- Sign in to work at Pacific View Regional Hospital for Period of Care 2. (*Note*: If you are already in the virtual hospital from a previous exercise, click on **Leave the Floor** and then on **Restart the Program** to get to the sign-in window.)
- From the Patient List, select Stacey Crider (Room 202).
- Click on **Go to Nurses' Station**.
- Click on **Chart** and then on **202**.
- Click on **History and Physical** and **Admissions**.

1. When was Stacey Crider's GDM diagnosed? How has it been managed up to this point?

2. Identify the risk factors for GDM.

3. Which risk factors for GDM are present in Stacey Crider?

4. What does Stacey Crider's physician suspect is the cause of her poorly controlled blood glucose levels?

- Click on **Physician's Orders**.

5. Look at Stacey Crider's admission orders. Write down the orders that are related to GDM.

6. Stacey Crider's physician ordered a hemoglobin A_{1c} test. What information will this test yield?
   a. The levels of blood glucose for the past 24 hours
   b. The amount of insulin needed to manage the pregnancy at the current gestation
   c. The degree of compliance with the prescribed therapeutic regimen
   d. The amount of dietary carbohydrates needed to maintain a healthy blood glucose level

On admission, Stacey Crider was in preterm labor. This was treated with magnesium sulfate tocolysis. She was also given a course of betamethasone.

• Click on **Return to Nurses' Station**.
• Click on the **Drug** icon in the lower left corner of the screen.
• Scroll down the drug list or use the search box to find betamethasone.

7. How might betamethasone affect Stacey Crider's GDM?

• Click on **Return to Nurses' Station**.
• Click on **Chart** and then on **202**.
• Click on **Physician's Notes** and review the note for Tuesday at 0700.

8. How does Stacey Crider's physician plan to deal with these potential medication effects?

Stacey Crider's other admission diagnosis was bacterial vaginosis.

• Click on **Return to Nurses' Station**.
• Click on **202** at the bottom of your screen.
• Click on **Patient Care** and then on **Nurse-Client Interactions**.
• Select and view the video titled **1115: Teaching—Diet, Infection**. (*Note:* Check the virtual clock to see whether enough time has elapsed. You can use the fast-forward feature to advance the time by 2-minute intervals if the video is not yet available. Then click again on **Patient Care** and **Nurse-Client Interactions** to refresh the screen.)

9. What is the relationship between Stacey Crider's bacterial vaginosis infection and her GDM?

Exercise 2

Virtual Hospital Activity

15 minutes

- Sign in to work at Pacific View Regional Hospital for Period of Care 1. (*Note*: If you are already in the virtual hospital from a previous exercise, click on **Leave the Floor** and then on **Restart the Program** to get to the sign-in window.)
- From the Patient List, select Stacey Crider (Room 202).
- Click on **Go to Nurses' Station**.

Stacey Crider needs her insulin so that she can eat breakfast. According to the MAR, she receives lispro insulin before each meal and NPH insulin at bedtime.

1. Based on your textbook reading, complete the table below.

Type of Insulin	Onset of Action	Peak	Duration
Lispro			
NPH			

- Click on **EPR** and then on **Login**.
- Select **202** from the Patient drop-down menu and **Vital Signs** from the Category drop-down menu.
- Look at the vital sign assessment documented on Wednesday at 0700.

2. What is Stacey Crider's blood glucose level?

- Click on **Exit EPR**.
- Click on **MAR**.
- Click on tab **202**.

3. What is Stacey Crider's prescribed insulin dosage?

- Click on **Return to Nurses' Station**.
- Click on **Chart** and then on **202**.
- Click on **Physician's Orders** and scroll to review the orders for Tuesday at 1900.

4. How much insulin should Stacey Crider receive? Why?

- Click on **Return to Nurses' Station**.
- Click on **Medication Room**.
- Click on **Unit Dosage** and then on drawer **202**.
- Click on **Insulin Lispro**.
- Click on **Put Medication on Tray** and then on **Close Drawer**.
- Click on **View Medication Room**.
- Click on **Preparation**.
- Click on **Prepare** next to Insulin Lispro and follow the prompts to complete the preparation of Stacey Crider's lispro insulin dose. Click on **Finish**.
- Click on **Return to Medication Room**.

You are almost ready to give Stacey Crider's insulin injection. However, before you do . . .

5. Considering lispro insulin's rapid onset of action, what else should you check before giving Stacey Crider her injection?

Now you're ready!

- Click on **202** at the bottom of the screen.
- Click on **Check Armband**.
- Click on **Patient Care** and then on **Medication Administration**.
- **Insulin Lispro** should be listed on the left side of your screen. Click on the down arrow next to Insulin Lispro and choose **Administer**.
- Follow the prompts to administer Stacey Crider's insulin injection. Indicate **Yes** to document the injection in the MAR.
- Click on **Leave the Floor**.
- Click on **Look at Your Preceptor's Evaluation**.
- Click on **Medication Scorecard**. How did you do?
- Click on **Return to Evaluations** and then on **Return to Menu**.

Exercise 3

Virtual Hospital Activity

30 minutes

- Sign in to work at Pacific View Regional Hospital for Period of Care 3. (*Note*: If you are already in the virtual hospital from a previous exercise, click on **Leave the Floor** and then on **Restart the Program** to get to the sign-in window.)
- From the Patient List, select Stacey Crider (Room 202).
- Click on **Go to Nurses' Station**.
- Click on **Chart** and then on **202**.
- Click on **Patient Education**.

Stacey Crider will likely be discharged home soon. Review her Patient Education record to determine her learning needs in regard to GDM.

1. List the educational goals for Stacey Crider regarding GDM.

Read the section on Care Management: Antepartum in your textbook.

2. Which of Stacey Crider's educational goals would apply to all women with GDM?

3. Which of Stacey Crider's educational goals would *not* apply to all women with GDM? Support your answer.

- Click on **Nurse's Notes** and scroll to the note for Wednesday at 0600.

4. How did the nurse describe Stacey Crider's ability to give her own insulin injection at that time?

- Click again on **Patient Education**.

5. What teaching has already been done with this patient on Wednesday in regard to GDM?

- Click on **Nurse's Notes** and review the note for 1200 Wednesday.

6. Do you think today's initial teaching on insulin administration was effective? Support your answer using objective documentation from the nurse's note.

Use the information you have obtained from the Patient Education form and the Nurse's Notes to answer the following questions.

7. Stacey Crider needs to know all of the following information. Which topic(s) would you choose to work on with her during this period of care? Select all that apply.

_____   Verbalize appropriate food choices and portions.

_____   Demonstrate good technique when administering insulin.

_____   Demonstrate good technique with self-monitoring of blood glucose.

_____   Recognize hyper- and hypoglycemia and how to treat each.

8. Give a rationale for your answer to question 7.

9. Which topic do you think Stacey Crider would *choose* to work on during this period of care? Select all that apply.

_____   Verbalize appropriate food choices and portions.

_____   Demonstrate good technique when administering insulin.

_____   Demonstrate good technique with self-monitoring of blood glucose.

_____   Recognize hyper- and hypoglycemia and how to treat each.

10. Give a rationale for your answer to question 9.

11. Stacey Crider is at an increased risk for developing glucose intolerance later in life. What advice would you give her to reduce this risk?

12. After delivery, what medical follow-up would you advise for Stacey Crider?

13. Could Stacey Crider's GDM affect her baby after birth? Explain.

12 _____

Medical-Surgical Disorders in Pregnancy

Reading Assignment: Medical-Surgical Disorders (Chapter 30)

Patients: Maggie Gardner, Room 204
Gabriela Valenzuela, Room 205

Goal: To demonstrate an understanding of the identification and management of selected medical-surgical problems in pregnancy.

Objectives:

• Identify appropriate interventions for managing selected medical-surgical problems in pregnancy.
• Plan and evaluate essential patient education during the acute phase of diagnosis.

Exercise 1

Virtual Hospital Activity

15 minutes

• Sign in to work at Pacific View Regional Hospital for Period of Care 1. (*Note*: If you are already in the virtual hospital from a previous exercise, click on **Leave the Floor** and then on **Restart the Program** to get to the sign-in window.)
• From the Patient List, select Gabriela Valenzuela (Room 205).
• Click on **Go to Nurses' Station**.
• Click on **Chart** and then on **205**.
• Click on **History and Physical**.

1. What does the physician note as Gabriela Valenzuela's cardiac problem?

2. _____ Mitral valve disease is one of the most common causes of cardiac disease in pregnant women. (True/False)

3. What cardiac symptoms has Gabriela Valenzuela experienced since becoming pregnant?

4. What manifestations, in addition to those that you identified in question 3, are associated with the condition? Select all that apply.

_____ Sharp pain in the right side of the chest

_____ Chest pain with rest

_____ Dyspnea with exertion

_____ Syncope

_____ Fluid retention

5. Why do pregnant women with cardiac disorders have problems during their pregnancies?

6. What abnormal assessment finding is noted in the History and Physical that would be associated with Gabriela Valenzuela's cardiac disorder?

Exercise 2

Virtual Hospital Activity

15 minutes

Autoimmune disorders encompass a wide variety of disorders that can be disruptive to the pregnancy process. Maggie Gardner has been admitted to rule out lupus. The following activities will explore the various aspects of this autoimmune disorder. First, review your textbook regarding systemic lupus erythematosus (SLE).

- Sign in to work at Pacific View Regional Hospital for Period of Care 2. (*Note*: If you are already in the virtual hospital from a previous exercise, click on **Leave the Floor** and then on **Restart the Program** to get to the sign-in window.)
- From the Patient List, select Maggie Gardner (Room 204).
- Click on **Go to Nurses' Station**.
- Click on **Chart** and then on **204**.
- Click on **History and Physical**.

1. Based on Maggie Gardner's History and Physical, what information would correlate with a diagnosis of SLE?

2. According to the textbook, disease activity at the beginning of pregnancy is an important predictor of

_____.

- Click on **Return to Nurses' Station**.
- Click on **204** at the bottom of the screen.
- Click on **Patient Care** and then on **Physical Assessment**.
- Perform a focused head-to-toe assessment by clicking on the various body system categories (yellow buttons) and body system subcategories (green buttons).

3. Based on your head-to-toe assessment, list four abnormal findings that are related to Maggie Gardner's diagnosis.

- Click on **Chart** and then on **204**.
- Click on **Patient Education**.

4. Based on your physical assessment, the information from the Patient Education section of the chart, and the fact that this is a new diagnosis, list three areas of teaching that need to be completed with this patient.

Exercise 3

Virtual Hospital Activity

20 minutes

- Sign in to work at Pacific View Regional Hospital for Period of Care 3. (*Note*: If you are already in the virtual hospital from a previous exercise, click on **Leave the Floor** and then on **Restart the Program** to get to the sign-in window.)
- From the Patient List, select Maggie Gardner (Room 204).
- Click on **Go to Nurses' Station**.
- Click on **Chart** and then on **204**.
- Click on the **Consultations** tab.
- Review the Rheumatology Consult.

1. List four things that the rheumatologist notes in her impressions regarding specific findings that are associated with a diagnosis of SLE for Maggie Gardner.

- Click on **Diagnostic Reports**.

2. Maggie Gardner had an ultrasound done before the consult with the rheumatologist. What were the findings as they relate to SLE? What were the follow-up recommendations?

3. What is the rheumatologist's plan regarding laboratory/diagnostics to gain a definitive diagnosis?

- Click on **Consultations** again.

4. According to the Rheumatology Consult, what is the plan regarding medications (immediate need)?

- Click on **Return to Nurses' Station**.
- Click on the **Drug** icon in the lower left corner of the screen.
- Find the Drug Guide profile of prednisone.

5. What patient education needs to be provided to Maggie Gardner regarding this medication?

- Click on **Return to Nurses' Station**.
- Click on **204** at the bottom of your screen.
- Click on **Patient Care** and then on **Nurse-Client Interactions**.
- Select and view the video titled **1530: Disease Management**. (*Note:* Check the virtual clock to see whether enough time has elapsed. You can use the fast-forward feature to advance the time by 2-minute intervals if the video is not yet available. Then click again on **Patient Care** and **Nurse-Client Interactions** to refresh the screen.)

6. During this video, the nurse provides Maggie Gardner with information regarding her disease. What two things does the nurse note that are important aspects of the patient's disease management during pregnancy?

7. What medication, ordered by the rheumatologist, will assist in the blood flow to the placenta? How?

8. Which of the following tests are likely to be implemented during a pregnancy complicated by SLE to assess fetal well-being? Select all that apply.

_____ Daily fetal movement counts

_____ Contraction stress testing weekly

_____ Ultrasound examinations

_____ Amniotic fluid volume assessment

_____ Assessment of progesterone levels

9. What key component does the nurse identify for Maggie Gardner that will assist in maintaining a healthy pregnancy?

- Click on **Chart** and then on **204**.
- Click on **Nursing Admission**.

10. What excuse does Maggie Gardner give for not keeping previous appointments with her doctor?

Exercise 4

Virtual Hospital Activity

15 minutes

- Sign in to work at Pacific View Regional Hospital for Period of Care 4. (*Note:* If you are already in the virtual hospital from a previous exercise, click on **Leave the Floor** and then on **Restart the Program** to get to the sign-in window.)
- From the Nurses' Station, click on **Chart** and then on **204**. (*Remember:* You are not able to visit patients or administer medications during Period of Care 4. You are able to review patient records only.)
- Click on **Laboratory Reports**.

1. The results are now available for the following laboratory tests that were ordered in Period of Care 2. What are the findings?

Laboratory Test	Result
C3	
C4	
CH50	
RPR	
ANA titer	
Anticardiolipin	
Anti-sm; Anti-DNA; Anti–SSA	
Anti-SSB	
Anti-RVV; Antiphospholipids	

- Click on **Consultations** and review the Rheumatology Consult.

2. The lab findings you recorded in question 1 are definitive for the diagnosis of SLE. According to the textbook and the Rheumatology Consult, what is the plan to manage this disease once the baby is delivered?

- Click on **Nurse's Notes.**

3. By Period of Care 4, Maggie Gardner has been provided with education regarding various aspects of her disease process, testing, and hospital procedures. Based on your review of the Nurse's Notes for Wednesday, what has she been specifically taught? Include the time each instruction took place.

4. Using correct NANDA nursing diagnosis terminology, write three possible nursing diagnoses for Maggie Gardner.

5. SLE requires long-term management because patients will experience remissions and exacerbations. What step did the rheumatologist take with Maggie Gardner to begin the long-term relationship that will be required to ensure a healthy outcome?

6. Which of the following risks may be noted as a result of Maggie Gardner's SLE? Select all that apply.

_____ HELLP syndrome

_____ Preeclampsia

_____ Premature rupture of membranes

_____ Preterm delivery

_____ Placental abruption

13

Mental Health Disorders and Substance Abuse

Reading Assignment: Mental Health Disorders and Substance Abuse (Chapter 31)
Acquired Problems of the Newborn (Chapter 34)

Patients: Kelly Brady, Room 203
Maggie Gardner, Room 204
Laura Wilson, Room 206

Goal: To demonstrate an understanding of the identification and management of selected mental health or substance abuse issues in pregnant women.

Objectives:

- Identify signs and symptoms of depression and anxiety in selected patients.
- Discuss the use of pharmacotherapy for treating depression and anxiety in pregnant and lactating patients.
- Assess and plan care for a substance-abusing woman with a term pregnancy.

Exercise 1

Virtual Hospital Activity

25 minutes

- Sign in to work at Pacific View Regional Hospital for Period of Care 1. (*Note*: If you are already in the virtual hospital from a previous exercise, click on **Leave the Floor** and then on **Restart the Program** to get to the sign-in window.)
- From the Patient List, select Kelly Brady (Room 203).
- Click on **Go to Nurses' Station**.

1. List signs and symptoms associated with major depression.

2. A nurse is caring for a pregnant woman who reports feelings of sadness and depression. Which of the following factors concerning depression in pregnancy should be understood by the nurse?
   a. Women who become depressed during pregnancy typically have a history of depression before pregnancy.
   b. The first trimester is the period of the pregnancy in which women will most likely develop depression.
   c. The childbearing years encompass the period of time in a woman's life in which depression and other mood disorders are most likely to occur.
   d. Depression is rare during pregnancy.

3. List risk factors for developing depression in pregnancy.

- Click on **Chart** and then on **203**.
- Click on **Mental Health** and review the record.

4. List Kelly Brady's signs/symptoms of major depression.

5. Does Kelly Brady meet the criteria for a diagnosis of major depression?

- Click on **Consultations** and review the Psychiatric Consult.

6. What risk factors are present in Kelly Brady that are associated with the development of major depression?

7. Using information from the Psychiatric Consult, list data that confirm the presence of the risk factors listed in question 6.

8. What is the management plan for Kelly Brady's depression recommended by the psychiatric consultant?

Read the section on Antidepressant Medications in your textbook.

9. What is the drug classification for paroxetine (Paxil)?

10. Kelly Brady plans to breastfeed her baby. How would you counsel her in regard to taking paroxetine (Paxil) while nursing?

11. What suggestions would you give Kelly Brady to help prevent the development of postpartum depression? (*Hint*: See the Teaching for Self-Management box in your textbook.)

Exercise 2

Virtual Hospital Activity

30 minutes

- Sign in to work at Pacific View Regional Hospital for Period of Care 1. (*Note*: If you are already in the virtual hospital from a previous exercise, click on **Leave the Floor** and then on **Restart the Program** to get to the sign-in window.)
- From the Patient List, select Maggie Gardner (Room 204).
- Click on **Go to Nurses' Station**.
- Click on **Chart** and then on **204**.
- Click on **Nursing Admission**.

1. What are Maggie Gardner's admission diagnoses?

2. What seems to be the major cause of Maggie Gardner's anxiety?

3. Is Maggie Gardner's anxiety currently affecting her lifestyle? Support your answer using data from the Nursing Admission.

- Click on **History and Physical**.
- Scroll to the OB History on page 2 of the History and Physical.

4. Below, list Maggie Gardner's obstetric history, using the GTPAL format.

   G:

   T:

   P:

   A:

   L:

5. Based on Maggie Gardner's previous pregnancy history, why do you think she might be especially anxious at this particular time in her pregnancy?

• Click on **Physician's Orders** and scroll to review the admission orders for Tuesday at 2115.

6. Identify the medication and dosage ordered specifically to treat Maggie Gardner's anxiety.

7. When providing education to Maggie Gardner concerning the use of buspirone, which of the following instructions should be included?
   a. Do not crush tablets.
   b. Administer with meals.
   c. Avoid grapefruit products.
   d. Reports of gastrointestinal upset are common with the medication.

8. Discuss the potential risks that may be associated with the use of buspirone during pregnancy.

• Click on **Return to Nurses' Station**.
• Click on **204** to go to the patient's room.
• Click on **Patient Care** and then on **Nurse-Client Interactions**.
• Select and view the video titled **0745: Evaluation—Efficacy of Drugs**. (*Note:* Check the virtual clock to see whether enough time has elapsed. You can use the fast-forward feature to advance the time by 2-minute intervals if the video is not yet available. Then click again on **Patient Care** and **Nurse-Client Interactions** to refresh the screen.)

9. How does Maggie Gardner describe her present emotional state?

- Click on the **Drug** icon in the lower left corner of the screen.
- Scroll down the drug list or use the search function to find buspirone.

10. Which of the following findings indicates the prescribed buspirone is having the desired effect in Maggie Gardner?
    a. Maggie Gardner sleeps soundly at night.
    b. Maggie Gardner reports feeling happier.
    c. Maggie Gardner appears less anxious.
    d. Maggie Gardner's emotions are less labile.

11. When providing education to Maggie Gardner concerning the time it will take for the buspirone to become effective, what information should be provided?
    a. Medication effects should be noticed in about 48 hours after starting the medication.
    b. Medication effects should be noticed a week after starting the medication.
    c. Medication effects should be noticed a month after starting the medication.
    d. Medication effects should be noticed about 3 weeks after starting the medication.

12. Is Maggie Gardner's buspirone dosage appropriate?

13. Scroll down to read the Patient Teaching section in the Drug Guide. Based on this information, do you agree with the nurse's explanation about buspirone's effectiveness in the 0745 video? If not, how would you counsel Maggie Gardner about the effectiveness of this medication?

Exercise 3

Virtual Hospital Activity

20 minutes

- Sign in to work at Pacific View Regional Hospital for Period of Care 2. (*Note*: If you are already in the virtual hospital from a previous exercise, click on **Leave the Floor** and then on **Restart the Program** to get to the sign-in window.)
- From the Patient List, select Laura Wilson (Room 206).
- Click on **Go to Nurses' Station**.
- Click on **Chart** and then on **206**.
- Click on **Nursing Admission**.

1. Complete the table below by documenting Laura Wilson's use of alcohol and recreational drugs based on your review of the Nursing Admission.

Substance	Reported Use
Tobacco	
Alcohol	
Marijuana	
Crack cocaine	

2. For each pregnancy-related risk listed in the table below, place an X under the substance(s) thought to be associated with that risk.

Pregnancy-Related Risk	Tobacco	Alcohol	Marijuana	Cocaine
Ectopic pregnancy				
Miscarriage				
Premature rupture of membranes				
Preterm birth				
Placenta previa				
Abruptio placentae				
IUGR				
Fetal alcohol spectrum disorder (FASD)				
IUFD/Stillbirth				
Long-term cognitive defects				
SIDS				
Fetal abnormalities				

- Click on **Return to Nurses' Station**.
- Click on **206** at the bottom of the screen.
- Click on **Patient Care** and then on **Nurse-Client Interactions**.
- Select and view the video titled **1115: Teaching—Effects of Drug Use**. (*Note:* Check the virtual clock to see whether enough time has elapsed. You can use the fast-forward feature to advance the time by 2-minute intervals if the video is not yet available. Then click again on **Patient Care** and **Nurse-Client Interactions** to refresh the screen.)

3. Does Laura Wilson consider herself to be addicted? Support your answer with comments from the video.

4. How does Laura Wilson think her drug use will affect her baby?

5. According to the nurse in the video, how might Laura Wilson's drug use affect the baby?

6. When confirming a diagnosis of fetal alcohol syndrome (FAS), manifestations must be present in which of the following categories? Select all that apply.

_____ Prenatal growth restriction

_____ Postnatal growth restriction

_____ Central nervous system malfunctions

_____ Musculoskeletal deformities

7. When caring for a woman who has been consuming alcohol during pregnancy, a nurse recognizes which of the following? Select all that apply.

_____ Neonates may experience alcohol withdrawal.

_____ In order for FAS to result, exposure to alcohol must have been present during each trimester.

_____ Exposure to higher amounts of alcohol is associated with more serious defects.

_____ The full picture of the damages of alcohol exposure may not be evident for years after the birth of the child.

_____ Girls account for the majority of newborns diagnosed with FAS.

8. Assume that you are the nurse caring for Laura Wilson today. Which interventions would be most appropriate to deal with Laura Wilson's substance abuse at this time? Select all that apply.

_____ Talking with Laura Wilson in a manner that conveys caring and concern

_____ Urging Laura Wilson to begin a drug treatment program today

_____ Explaining to Laura Wilson that she may lose custody of her baby if her drug use continues

_____ Involving other members of the health care team in Laura Wilson's care

9. Explain your choice(s) in question 8.

Labor and Birth Complications

Reading Assignment: Labor and Birth Complications (Chapter 32)

Patients: Dorothy Grant, Room 201
Stacey Crider, Room 202
Kelly Brady, Room 203
Gabriela Valenzuela, Room 205

Goal: To demonstrate an understanding of the identification and management of selected labor and birth complications.

Objectives:

- Assess and identify signs and symptoms present in the patient with preterm labor.
- Describe appropriate nursing care for the patient in preterm labor.
- Develop a birth plan to meet the needs of the preterm infant.

Exercise 1

Virtual Hospital Activity

20 minutes

- Sign in to work at Pacific View Regional Hospital for Period of Care 2. (*Note*: If you are already in the virtual hospital from a previous exercise, click on **Leave the Floor** and then on **Restart the Program** to get to the sign-in window.)
- From the Patient List, select Dorothy Grant (Room 201) and Gabriela Valenzuela (Room 205).
- Click on **Go to Nurses' Station**.
- Click on **Chart** and then on **201**.
- Click on **History and Physical**.

1. Using the information found in the History and Physical, complete the table below for Dorothy Grant.

Patient	Weeks of Gestation	Reason for Admission
Dorothy Grant		

- Click on **Return to Nurses' Station**.
- Click again on **Chart**; this time, click on **205**.
- Click on **History and Physical**.

2. Using the information found in the History and Physical, complete the table below for Gabriela Valenzuela.

Patient	Weeks of Gestation	Reason for Admission
Gabriela Valenzuela		

- Click on **Return to Nurses' Station**.
- Click on **201** at the bottom of the screen.
- Click on **Patient Care** and then on **Physical Assessment**.
- Click on **Pelvic** and then on **Reproductive**.

3. Complete the table below with the results of Dorothy Grant's initial cervical examination.

Patient	Time	Dilation	Effacement	Station
Dorothy Grant				

- Click on **205** at the bottom of the screen to go to Gabriela Valenzuela's room.
- Click on **Patient Care** and then on **Physical Assessment**.
- Click on **Pelvic** and then on **Reproductive**.

4. Record the results of Gabriela Valenzuela's initial cervical examination in the table below.

Patient	Time	Dilation	Effacement	Station
Gabriela Valenzuela				

Read the section on Early Recognition and Diagnosis of preterm labor in your textbook.

5. What criteria are necessary in order to make a diagnosis of preterm labor?

6. As of Wednesday at 0800, would you consider either or both of these patients to be in preterm labor? Give a rationale for your answer.

Read the section on Suppression of Uterine Activity in your textbook to answer the following questions.

7. Would you recommend tocolytic therapy for Gabriela Valenzuela? Support your answer.

8. Match each of the medications below with the corresponding mechanism of action. Mechanisms of action may be used more than once.

Medication

_____ Magnesium sulfate

_____ Nifedipine (Procardia)

_____ Terbutaline (Brethine)

_____ Indomethacin (Indocin)

Mechanism of Action

a. Inhibits calcium from entering smooth muscle cells, thus relaxing uterine contractions

b. Relaxes uterine smooth muscle as a result of stimulation of beta$_2$ receptors on uterine smooth muscle

c. CNS depressant; promotes relaxation of smooth muscles

d. Suppresses preterm labor by blocking the production of prostaglandins

Exercise 2

Virtual Hospital Activity

30 minutes

• Sign in to work at Pacific View Regional Hospital for Period of Care 1. (*Note*: If you are already in the virtual hospital from a previous exercise, click on **Leave the Floor** and then on **Restart the Program** to get to the sign-in window.)
• From the Patient List, select Stacey Crider (Room 202).
• Click on **Get Report**.

Stacey Crider was admitted yesterday in preterm labor and placed on magnesium sulfate. Her other admission diagnoses were bacterial vaginosis and gestational diabetes mellitus with poorly controlled blood glucose levels.

1. What is Stacey Crider's current status in regard to preterm labor?

- Click on **Go to Nurses' Station**.
- Click on **Chart** and then on **202**.
- Click on **Physician's Orders** and scroll to review the orders for Wednesday at 0715.

2. Which of these orders relate specifically to Stacey Crider's diagnosis of preterm labor?

- Still in the Physician's Orders, scroll to review the orders for Wednesday at 0730.

3. What medication changes are ordered?

Read about terbutaline and nifedipine in Tocolytic Therapy for Preterm Labor in your textbook.

4. Why do you think Stacey Crider's physician changed his orders so quickly?

- Click on **Return to Nurses' Station**.
- Click on **202** at the bottom of the screen.
- Click on **Take Vital Signs**.

5. What are Stacey Crider's vital signs at 0800?

Temperature

Heart rate

Respirations

Blood pressure

6. When administering nifedipine, which of the following side effects is associated with the medication and would warrant holding the dose pending notification of the physician?
   a. Hypertension
   b. Tachycardia
   c. Bradycardia
   d. Hypotension

7. Which vital sign parameters provide the most important information you would need before giving Stacey Crider's nifedipine dose? Why?

Like Dorothy Grant and Kelly Brady, Stacey Crider is also receiving betamethasone. Read about Promotion of Fetal Lung Maturity in your textbook and then answer the following questions.

8. Why are all three of these patients receiving antenatal corticosteroid therapy?

9. What other benefits does this class of medication provide for preterm infants?

- Click on **MAR**.
- Click on tab **202**.

10. What is Stacey Crider's ordered betamethasone dosage?

11. How does this dosage compare with the recommended dosage listed in the section on Antenatal Glucocorticoid Therapy with Betamethasone or Dexamethasone Medication Guide in your textbook?

- Click on **Return to Room 202**.
- Click on **Medication Room**.
- Click on **Unit Dosage** and then on drawer **202**.
- Click on **Betamethasone**.

- Click on **Put Medication on Tray** and then on **Close Drawer**.
- Click on **View Medication Room**.
- Click on **Preparation**.
- Click on **Prepare** next to Betamethasone and follow the Preparation Wizard's prompts to complete preparation of Stacey Crider's betamethasone dose.
- Click on **Return to Medication Room**.
- Click on **202** at the bottom of the screen.
- Click on **Check Armband** and then on **Check Allergies**.
- Click on **Patient Care** and then on **Medication Administration**.
- Find Betamethasone listed on the left side of your screen. Click on the down arrow next to **Select** and choose **Administer**.
- Follow the Administration Wizard's prompts to administer Stacey Crider's betamethasone injection. Indicate **Yes** to document the injection in the MAR.
- Click on **Leave the Floor**.
- Click on **Look at Your Preceptor's Evaluation**.
- Click on **Medication Scorecard**. How did you do?
- Click on **Return to Evaluation** and then on **Return to Menu**.

Exercise 3

Virtual Hospital Activity

20 minutes

- Sign in to work at Pacific View Regional Hospital for Period of Care 4. (*Note*: If you are already in the virtual hospital from a previous exercise, click on **Leave the Floor** and then on **Restart the Program** to get to the sign-in window.)
- Click on **Chart** and then on **201**. (*Remember:* You are not able to visit patients or administer medications during Period of Care 4. You are able to review patient records only.)
- Click on **Nurse's Notes** and scroll to review the note for Wednesday 1815.

1. Despite receiving terbutaline for tocolysis, Dorothy Grant's labor continues to progress. What are the findings from her cervical examination at this time?

- Scroll to the note for Wednesday 1840. It states that Dorothy Grant is being prepped for delivery.

2. If you were the nurse caring for Dorothy Grant during delivery, what special preparations would you make to care for the baby immediately after birth?

- Click on **Return to Nurses' Station**.
- Click on **Chart** and then on **205**.
- Click on **Physician's Notes** and scroll to review the note for Wednesday at 0800.

3. What is the anticipated outcome of Gabriela Valenzuela's labor, according to this note?

- Still in the Physician's Notes, scroll to review the notes for Wednesday at 1415 and 1455.

4. What preparations have been made during the day for the birth of Gabriela Valenzuela's baby?

Read the information on Cesarean Birth found in your textbook.

Kelly Brady was admitted yesterday with severe preeclampsia at 26 weeks of gestation. Her preeclampsia is now worsening.

5. Why does Kelly Brady's physician now recommend immediate delivery?

6. What general risks related to cesarean birth does Kelly Brady's physician discuss with her?

7. Because of Kelly Brady's early gestational age (26 weeks), her physician anticipates a classical uterine incision. How will this type of incision affect Kelly Brady's birth options in future pregnancies?

- Click on **Physician's Orders** and scroll to review the orders for Wednesday 1540.

8. List the orders to be carried out before Kelly Brady's surgery. State the purpose of each.

Order	Purpose

9. Can you think of other common preoperative procedures? List them below. (*Hint*: Refer to a basic Medical-Surgical textbook for ideas if you need help!)

LESSON 15

Newborn Complications

Reading Assignment: Acquired Problems of the Newborn (Chapter 34)

Nursing Care of the High Risk Newborn and Family (Chapter 36)

Patients: Stacey Crider, Room 202

Kelly Brady, Room 203

Gabriela Valenzuela, Room 205

Laura Wilson, Room 206

Goal: To demonstrate an understanding of the identification and management of selected common complications of newborns.

Objectives:

- Describe commonly occurring problems of infants of mothers with diabetes.
- List nursing interventions related to hypoglycemia in infants of mothers with diabetes.
- Identify risk factors for development of early-onset group B streptococci (GBS) infection and human immunodeficiency virus (HIV).
- Describe common signs and symptoms of early-onset GBS infection.
- List nursing interventions for preventing the transmission of HIV to the neonate.
- Identify signs and symptoms of in utero drug exposure in the neonate.
- Identify common problems found in extremely low-birth-weight infants.

Exercise 1

Virtual Hospital Activity

15 minutes

- Sign in to work at Pacific View Regional Hospital for Period of Care 4. (*Note*: If you are already in the virtual hospital from a previous exercise, click on **Leave the Floor** and then on **Restart the Program** to get to the sign-in window.)
- Click on **Chart** and then on **202**. (*Remember:* You are not able to visit patients or administer medications during Period of Care 4. You are able to review patient records only.)
- Click on **History and Physical**.

1. When was Stacey Crider's gestational diabetes mellitus (GDM) diagnosed?

2. How was Stacey Crider's GDM managed?

- Click on **Nursing Admission**.

3. What was the status of Stacey Crider's GDM when she was admitted to the hospital at 27 weeks of gestation?

Assume that Stacey Crider has given birth and you are now the nurse caring for her baby. Read the section on Infants of Mothers with Diabetes in your textbook.

4. Listed below are problems often seen in infants of mothers with diabetes. For each problem, identify the mechanism(s) responsible for that complication by writing the corresponding letter(s) in the blank. Mechanisms may be used more than once.

Problems	Responsible Mechanisms
_____ Congenital anomalies	a. Episodes of ketoacidosis
_____ Macrosomia	b. Fetal hyperinsulinemia
_____ Hypoglycemia	c. Maternal hyperglycemia
_____ Small-for-gestational-age (SGA) infant	d. Fluctuations in maternal blood glucose levels
_____ Respiratory distress syndrome	e. Maternal severe vascular disease

5. The nurse caring for Stacey Crider's infant knows that hypoglycemia in the term infant is recognized as:
   a. a blood glucose level less than 35 mg/dL.
   b. a blood glucose level less than 40 mg/dL.
   c. a blood glucose level less than 45 mg/dL.
   d. a blood glucose level less than 50 mg/dL.

6. The nurse caring for the infant at risk for hypoglycemia recognizes which of the following to be manifestations of hypoglycemia? Select all that apply.

   _____ Bradycardia

   _____ Hypotension

   _____ Jitteriness

   _____ Apnea

   _____ Tachypnea

   _____ Cyanosis

   _____ Warm, flushed skin

7. List four nursing interventions that can be implemented to prevent or manage hypoglycemia in Stacey Crider's baby.

Exercise 2

Virtual Hospital Activity

30 minutes

Gabriela Valenzuela was admitted at 34 weeks of gestation with vaginal bleeding and uterine contractions following a motor vehicle accident (MVA). Her labor progressed throughout the day on Wednesday, and vaginal delivery is expected.

- Sign in to work at Pacific View Regional Hospital for Period of Care 4. (*Note*: If you are already in the virtual hospital from a previous exercise, click on **Leave the Floor** and then on **Restart the Program** to get to the sign-in window.)
- Click on **MAR** and then on tab **205** for Gabriela Valenzuela's records. (*Remember:* You are not able to visit patients or administer medications during Period of Care 4. You are able to review patient records only.)

1. What medication has Gabriela Valenzuela been receiving for GBS prophylaxis today?

* Click on **Return to Nurses' Station**.
* Click on **Chart** and then on **205**.
* Click on **Nurse's Notes** and scroll to review the note for Wednesday at 1820.

2. What are the findings of Gabriela Valenzuela's cervical examination at this time?

3. Listed below are risk factors for the development of early-onset GBS infection. Place an X beside the risk factor that you know would apply to Gabriela Valenzuela's baby.

_____ Low birth weight

_____ Preterm birth

_____ Rupture of membranes of more than 18 hours

_____ Maternal fever

_____ Previous infant with GBS infection

_____ Maternal GBS bacteriuria

_____ Multiple gestation

4. Early-onset GBS infection most commonly manifests _____.

Early-onset GBS infection usually results from _____ transmission from the

_____.

5. If you were the nurse caring for Gabriela Valenzuela's baby, what signs/symptoms might you see if the baby developed early-onset GBS?

Laura Wilson is a gravida 1 para 0 at 37 weeks of gestation who is also HIV-positive. She was admitted last night with fever, vomiting, and diarrhea to rule out acute abdomen and pyelonephritis. During the day on Wednesday, Laura Wilson began having mild uterine contractions.

* Click on **Return to Nurses' Station**.
* Click on **Chart** and then on **206**.
* Click on **Physician's Notes** and review the note for Wednesday at 0830.

6. Below, record Laura Wilson's HIV-related lab values.

CD4 count

HIV 1 RNA count

• Click on **Physician's Orders** and scroll to review the admission orders for Tuesday at 2130.

7. What is Laura Wilson's current antiretroviral drug regimen?

• Click on **Nurse's Notes** and scroll to review the note for Wednesday at 1830.

8. What event occurred at 1815?

9. Is Laura Wilson in labor at this time? Support your answer.

10. List factors that, if present, would decrease the risk for transmission of HIV to Laura Wilson's baby during the birth process. Which risk factor does Laura Wilson have at this time?

11. All infants born to seropositive mothers should be assumed to be _____. The accuracy of

HIV testing in infants varies according to the _____ and is dependent on

_____.

12. What are the current testing recommendations for diagnosing HIV infection in newborns?

13. Assume that you are the nurse caring for Laura Wilson's baby in the newborn nursery. List nursing interventions to decrease risk for viral transmission to the baby.

Exercise 3

Virtual Hospital Activity

10 minutes

In addition to being HIV-positive, Laura Wilson also has a past and current history of substance abuse.

- Sign in to work at Pacific View Regional Hospital for Period of Care 4. (*Note*: If you are already in the virtual hospital from a previous exercise, click on **Leave the Floor** and then on **Restart the Program** to get to the sign-in window.)
- Click on **Chart** and then on **206** for Laura Wilson's chart. (*Remember:* You are not able to visit patients or administer medications during Period of Care 4. You are able to review patient records only.)
- Click on **Nursing Admission**.

1. Complete the chart below with information on Laura Wilson's current use of alcohol and recreational drugs.

Substance	Reported Use
Alcohol	
Marijuana	
Crack cocaine	

Read about alcohol, marijuana, and cocaine in the Substance Abuse section in your textbook.

2. Listed below are problems often seen in infants exposed prenatally to alcohol, marijuana, or cocaine. Indicate the substance(s) thought to be associated with each problem by marking an X in the proper column(s). More than one drug may be associated with each problem.

Problem	Alcohol	Marijuana	Cocaine
Craniofacial abnormalities			
Intrauterine growth restriction (IUGR)			
Hyperactivity			
Congenital anomalies			
Developmental delay			
Hypersensitivity to noise and external stimuli			
Neurologic/cognitive/ behavioral effects			

3. A diagnosis of fetal alcohol syndrome (FAS) is based on minimal criteria of signs in each of three

   categories: _____, _____,

   and _____. A baby who has been affected by prenatal exposure to alcohol

   but does not meet the criteria for FAS may be said to have an _____ or

   _____.

Read the Nursing Care section in your textbook.

4. List several appropriate interventions for the nurse assigned to work with Laura Wilson as she learns to accept and care for her drug-exposed baby.

Exercise 4

Virtual Hospital Activity

20 minutes

Kelly Brady was admitted with severe preeclampsia at 26 weeks of gestation. Because of worsening maternal condition, she gives birth via cesarean on Wednesday.

- Sign in to work at Pacific View Regional Hospital for Period of Care 4. (*Note*: If you are already in the virtual hospital from a previous exercise, click on **Leave the Floor** and then on **Restart the Program** to get to the sign-in window.)
- Click on **Chart** and then on **203** for Kelly Brady's chart. (*Remember:* You are not able to visit patients or administer medications during Period of Care 4. You are able to review patient records only.)
- Click on **Diagnostic Reports**.

1. According to the ultrasound done on Tuesday, what is Kelly Brady's baby's estimated fetal weight?

- Click on **Consultations**.
- Review the Neonatology Consult for Wednesday at 0800.

2. List common problems for babies born at 26 weeks of gestation at Pacific View Regional Hospital, according to the neonatologist who met with Kelly Brady and her husband.

Read the section on Preterm Infants in your textbook.

3. If Kelly Brady's baby's actual weight is close to her estimated weight, in which weight category will she be placed? Why?

4. Many body systems or functions are likely to be impaired in very-low-birth-weight (VLBW) infants. Which of the following systems or functions were addressed by the neonatologist in his consultation with Kelly Brady? Select all that apply.

_____ Respiratory function

_____ Cardiovascular function

_____ Maintenance of body temperature

_____ Central nervous system (CNS) function

_____ Maintenance of adequate nutrition

_____ Maintenance of renal function

_____ Maintenance of hematologic status

_____ Resistance to infection

Read the section on Parental Adaptation to Preterm Infant in your textbook.

5. List several psychological tasks that Kelly Brady and/or her husband must accomplish as parents of Baby Brady.

6. Write a nursing diagnosis appropriate for the Bradys, as parents of a premature baby who will have an extended neonatal intensive care unit (NICU) stay.

7. List several nursing interventions to assist the Bradys in accomplishing the parenting tasks listed in question 5.

16

Perinatal Loss, Bereavement, and Grief

Reading Assignment: Perinatal Loss, Bereavement, and Grief (Chapter 37)

Patient: Maggie Gardner, Room 204

Goal: To demonstrate an understanding of the grieving process and how it relates to coping with a current pregnancy.

Objectives:

- Identify the various types of loss as they relate to a pregnancy.
- Describe the stages and phases of the grieving process.
- Identify various methods of coping exhibited by patients who have experienced the loss of a newborn.

Exercise 1

Writing Activity

10 minutes

1. Parents may grieve not only the death of a newborn, but also the birth of a baby with a

   _____.

2. List other times that couples may grieve a loss related to pregnancy.

3. What type of effects do women experience if a pregnancy ends early as a result of miscarriage?

4. Premature birth occurs in approximately what percentage of pregnancies?
    a. 7.5%
    b. 11.5%
    c. 17.5%
    d. 22.5%

5. Grief is _____, is a _____, is _____, and is

    _____.

6. _____ All women and men who undergo a loss receive the support that they need. (True/False)

Exercise 2

Virtual Hospital Activity

10 minutes

- Sign in to work at Pacific View Regional Hospital for Period of Care 4. (*Note*: If you are already in the virtual hospital from a previous exercise, click on **Leave the Floor** and then on **Restart the Program** to get to the sign-in window.)
- Click on **Chart** and then on **204** for Maggie Gardner's chart. (*Remember:* You are not able to visit patients or administer medications during Period of Care 4. You are able to review patient records only.)
- Review the **History and Physical**.

1. How many losses related to pregnancy has Maggie Gardner experienced?

- Click on the **Nursing Admission**.

2. What is the evidence that Maggie Gardner's previous losses are affecting her current pregnancy and care?

- Click on the **Consultations** tab and review the Pastoral Consult.

3. To what does Maggie Gardner attribute her inability to have a child?

4. List three therapeutic measures the chaplain can use to assist Maggie Gardner through these feelings as part of her grieving process?

5. What did the chaplain accomplish during his time with Maggie Gardner?

Exercise 3

Virtual Hospital Activity

15 minutes

1. What is grief?

2. What are the three phases of grief?

3. Within the phases of grief, what are the tasks of grief?

4. Mothers are the focus during the loss of an infant; however, the _____ shares the

_____ level of grief.

5. List the emotions that are experienced during the time period of intense grief.

6. What question do patients most commonly ask during the phase of reorganization? Explain.

- Sign in to work at Pacific View Regional Hospital for Period of Care 4. (*Note:* If you are already in the virtual hospital from a previous exercise, click on **Leave the Floor** and then on **Restart the Program** to get to the sign-in window.)
- Click on **Chart** and then on **204**. (*Remember:* You are not able to visit patients or administer medications during Period of Care 4. You are able to review patient records only.)
- Review the **History and Physical**.

7. What correlation do you see between the information in Maggie Gardner's History and Physical and the information presented in the Reorganization section in your textbook?

- Click on **Consultations** and review the Pastoral Care Spiritual Assessment.

8. Culture and religion play very large roles in how individuals handle a loss. How has Maggie Gardner handled her losses?

LESSON **17**

Medication Administration

Reading Assignment: Nursing Care of the Family During the Postpartum Period (Chapter 21)

Patients: Dorothy Grant, Room 201
Stacey Crider, Room 202
Maggie Gardner, Room 204
Laura Wilson, Room 206

Goal: To correctly administer selected medications to obstetric patients.

Objective:

- Correctly administer selected medications to obstetric patients, observing the Six Rights.

Exercise 1

Virtual Hospital Activity

20 minutes

Dorothy Grant was admitted at 30 weeks of gestation for observation following blunt abdominal trauma. She is bleeding vaginally and may have sustained a placental abruption. Your assignment for this exercise is to give Rh immune globulin to Dorothy Grant.

- Sign in to work at Pacific View Regional Hospital for Period of Care 2. (*Note*: If you are already in the virtual hospital from a previous exercise, click on **Leave the Floor** and then on **Restart the Program** to get to the sign-in window.)
- From the Patient List, select Dorothy Grant (Room 201).

Read about Rh immune globulin in your textbook.

1. Rh immune globulin is a solution of _____ that contains _____.

   Rh immune globulin is given to _____

   who has had a _____.

   Rh immune globulin prevents sensitization by _____

   _____.

2. Listed below are reasons that Rh immune globulin might be administered. Why has it been ordered for Dorothy Grant?
   a. Within 72 hours of giving birth to an Rh-positive infant
   b. Prophylactically at 28 weeks of gestation
   c. Following an incident or exposure risk that occurs after 28 weeks of gestation
   d. During first trimester pregnancy following miscarriage or elective abortion or ectopic pregnancy

3. List the information about Dorothy Grant that must be determined before giving her Rh immune globulin.

- Click on **Go to Nurses' Station**.
- Click on **Chart** and then on **201**.
- Click on **Physician's Orders** and review the orders for Wednesday at 0730.

4. Write the physician's order for Rh immune globulin.

5. According to your textbook, is this the correct dosage and route?

- Click on **Laboratory Reports**.
- Locate the results for 0245 Wednesday.
- Scroll down to find the type and screen results.

6. Dorothy Grant's blood type is _____.

7. What additional information do you need? Why? Is that information available?

- Click on **Return to Nurses' Station**.
- Click on **Medication Room**.
- Click on **Refrigerator** and then click on the refrigerator door to open it.
- Click on **Rho(D) Immune Globulin**.
- Click on **Put Medication on Tray** and then on **Close Door**.
- Click on **View Medication Room**.
- Click on **Preparation**.
- Click on **Prepare** next to Rho(D) Immune Globulin and follow the prompts to complete preparation of this medication.
- Click on **Return to Medication Room**.
- Click on **201** at the bottom of the screen.
- Click on **Check Armband**.
- Click on **Patient Care** and then on **Medication Administration**.

You are almost ready to give Dorothy Grant's injection. However, before you do . . .

8. _____ Rh immune globulin is often considered a blood product. (True/False)

9. Suppose Dorothy Grant tells you that because of her religious beliefs, she absolutely refuses to accept blood or blood products. How would you handle the situation?

Now you're ready to administer the medication!

- Click on the down arrow next to **Select**; choose **Administer**.
- Follow the prompts to administer Dorothy Grant's injection. Indicate **Yes** to document the injection in the MAR.
- Click on **Leave the Floor**.
- Click on **Look at Your Preceptor's Evaluation**.
- Click on **Medication Scorecard**. How did you do?
- Click on **Return to Evaluation** and then on **Return to Menu**.

Exercise 2

Virtual Hospital Activity

10 minutes

- Sign in to work at Pacific View Regional Hospital for Period of Care 1. (*Note*: If you are already in the virtual hospital from a previous exercise, click on **Leave the Floor** and then on **Restart the Program** to get to the sign-in window.)
- From the Patient List, select Maggie Gardner (Room 204).
- Click on **Go to Nurses' Station**.
- Click on the **Chart** and then on **204**.
- Click on the **Nursing Admission**.

1. Maggie Gardner repeatedly verbalizes anxiety throughout the Nursing Admission. What is her primary concern? Why?

2. Maggie Gardner states that before this pregnancy she had a highly adaptive coping mechanism. How does she consider her ability to cope at this point? Why?

- Click on the **Physician's Orders**.

3. What medication has the physician ordered to help Maggie Gardner with her anxiety?

- Click on **Return to Nurses' Station**.
- Click on the **Drug** icon in the lower-left corner of your screen.
- Use the search box or the scroll bar to find the medication you identified in question 3.
- Review all of the information provided regarding this drug.

4. What is the mechanism of action for this drug?

- Click on **Return to Nurses' Station**.
- Click on **204** at the bottom of the screen.
- Click on **Patient Care** and then on **Nurse-Client Interaction**.
- Select and view the video titled **0745: Evaluation—Efficacy of Drugs**. (*Note:* Check the virtual clock to see whether enough time has elapsed. You can use the fast-forward feature to advance the time by 2-minute intervals if the video is not yet available. Then click again on **Patient Care** and **Nurse-Client Interactions** to refresh the screen.)

5. According to the nurse, how long will it take for Maggie Gardner to see therapeutic effects? How does this correlate with what was found when reviewing the Teaching Section of the Drug Guide?

Exercise 3

Virtual Hospital Activity

10 minutes

In this exercise, you will administer betamethasone to Stacey Crider, who was admitted to the hospital at 27 weeks of gestation in preterm labor.

- Sign in to work at Pacific View Regional Hospital for Period of Care 1. (*Note*: If you are already in the virtual hospital from a previous exercise, click on **Leave the Floor** and then on **Restart the Program** to get to the sign-in window.)
- From the Patient List, select Stacey Crider (Room 202).

1. Before preparing Stacey Crider's betamethasone, what do you need to do first?

- Click on **Go to Nurses' Station**.
- Click on **Chart** and then on **202**.
- Click on **Physician's Orders** and scroll until you find the order for betamethasone.

2. After verifying the physician's order, what is your next step?

- Click on **Return to Nurses' Station**.
- Click on **Medication Room**.
- Click on **Unit Dosage** and then on drawer **202**.
- Click on **Betamethasone**.
- Click on **Put Medication on Tray** and then on **Close Drawer**.
- Click on **View Medication Room**.
- Click on **Preparation**.
- Click on **Prepare** next to Betamethasone and follow the prompts to complete preparation of Stacey Crider's betamethasone dose. When the preparation of this medication is completed, click on **Finish**.
- Click on **Return to Medication Room**.

3. Now that the medication is prepared, what is your next step?

- Click on **202** at the bottom of the screen.
- Click on **Check Armband** and then on **Check Allergies**.
- Click on **Patient Care** and then on **Medication Administration**.
- Click on the down arrow next to Select and choose **Administer**.
- Follow the prompts to administer Stacey Crider's betamethasone injection.

4. What's the final step in the process?

- If you haven't already, indicate **Yes** to document the injection in the MAR.
- Click on **Leave the Floor**.
- Click on **Look at Your Preceptor's Evaluation**.
- Click on **Medication Scorecard**. How did you do?
- Click on **Return to Evaluation** and then on **Return to Menu**.

Exercise 4

Virtual Hospital Activity

15 minutes

- Sign in to work at Pacific View Regional Hospital for Period of Care 1. (*Note*: If you are already in the virtual hospital from a previous exercise, click on **Leave the Floor** and then on **Restart the Program** to get to the sign-in window.)
- From the Patient List, select Laura Wilson (Room 206).
- Click on **Go to Nurses' Station**.
- Click on **MAR**.
- Click on tab **206**.

1. Laura Wilson's medications for Wednesday include several different types of drugs. Which of the following medications does she take because she has human immunodeficiency virus (HIV)?
   a. Zidovudine 200 mg PO every 8 hours
   b. Prenatal multivitamin 1 tablet PO daily
   c. Lactated Ringer's 1000 mL IV continuous

- Click on **Return to Nurses' Station**.
- Click on the **Drug** icon in the lower-left corner of the screen.
- Use the search box or the scroll bar to find the drug you identified in question 1.

2. What is the mechanism of action for this drug?

3. What is the drug's therapeutic effect?

4. Does this medication cross the placenta? Is it distributed in breast milk?

5. What symptoms/side effects of this medication need to be reported to the physician?

6. How should this medication be taken?

7. As a final assignment, you are to give Laura Wilson the medication that is due at 0800. During these lessons, we have provided you with the detailed instructions on how to give medications. Now it is time for you to fly solo. If you are administering the medication from the last question, start by clicking on **Return to Nurses' Station**. Don't forget the Six Rights of medication administration . . . and have fun!! Below, document how you did.

If you'd like to get more practice, there are other medications that can be given at the beginning of the first three periods of care. Below is a list of the patients, the medications, the routes of administration, and the administration times you can use. As you practice, be sure to select the correct patient when you sign in so that you can get a Medication Scorecard for evaluation after you prepare and administer a medication.

PERIOD OF CARE 1

Room 201, Dorothy Grant

0730/0800

Betamethasone 12 mg IM

Prenatal multivitamin PO

Room 202, Stacey Crider

0800

Prenatal multivitamin PO

Metronidazole 500 mg PO

Betamethasone 12 mg IM

Insulin lispro subQ

Nifedipine 20 mg PO

Room 203, Kelly Brady

0730/0800

Prenatal multivitamin PO

Ferrous sulfate 325 mg PO

Labetalol hydrochloride 400 mg PO

Nifedipine 10 mg PO

Room 204, Maggie Gardner

0800

Prenatal multivitamin PO

Buspirone hydrochloride 5 mg PO

Room 205, Gabriela Valenzuela

0800

Ampicillin 2 g IV

Betamethasone 12 mg IM

Room 206, Laura Wilson

0800

Zidovudine 200 mg PO

Prenatal multivitamin PO

PERIOD OF CARE 2

Room 201, Dorothy Grant

1200

Rh immune globulin IM

Room 202, Stacey Crider

1200

Insulin lispro subQ

Room 203, Kelly Brady

1130

Betamethasone 12 mg IM

Room 204, Maggie Gardner

1115

Prednisone 40 mg PO

Aspirin 81 mg PO

PERIOD OF CARE 3

Room 204, Maggie Gardner

1500

Buspirone hydrochloride 5 mg PO